Narcissistic Child

Mothers and Fathers Who Do
Co-Parenting, Look Out for
Behavior Signs in Your Children
and Understand the Covert
Narcissistic Personality Disorder

Mona Diggins

Table of Contents

Introduction

A child who is allowed to be disrespectful to his parents will not have true respect for anyone.

—Bill Graham

Narcissism. It's an issue that is becoming more and more visible in our popular culture. We tend to say that someone who is particularly vain or self-absorbed is "narcissistic." Many of us were raised with the legend of Narcissus, the Greek hero who falls hopelessly in love with his own reflection. Pop and parapsychology titles increasingly cite the dangers of dating narcissists, warning their readers that narcissism belongs on the "dark triad" of personality types and exhibiting terrifying examples of narcissism in dangerous people like serial killers or dictators.

But from a clinical perspective, "narcissism" means much, much more than vanity or selfishness. While it can be a dangerous and destructive force in a person's life, narcissistic personality disorder does not necessarily make someone a serial killer or an abuser. The realities behind this mental condition are as complex as any other personality disorder, and popular misunderstanding of narcissism only makes the world more dangerous for both the people who fall victim to the darker manifestations of this personality type, as well as for narcissists themselves.

Like all personality disorders, narcissism begins in early childhood and is partly created by certain conditions experienced at this phase of life. This book will help to demystify this most misunderstood of personality disorders. It will provide clear, easy-to-read explanations of what narcissism is and how it manifests in young children. As a parent or guardian of a young child, you can use the information in this book to determine whether or not your child is displaying the early warning signs of this disorder and subsequently get your child the professional help they need before the disorder spins out of control. In this book, you will find clinically-sanctioned guidance on how to manage children with narcissistic personality disorder in ways that protect you, your child, and the other children around them.

Most parents worry for their children and do their best to ensure that they grow up as happily and healthily as possible. An increasingly difficult relationship with your child does not necessarily mean that they have narcissism or any other personality disorder. However, if your child does have a personality disorder, this is no more cause for concern than any other kind of diagnosis your child may receive. Children diagnosed with everything from bipolar disorder to autism grow up to be happy, fulfilled, and well-adjusted adults, and narcissistic personality disorder is not different. The important thing for you is to learn as much as you can about what causes this disorder so that you can prevent it from further developing in a child who is displaying its warning signs. If your child is already showing advanced symptoms of the disorder, it's equally important for you to get your child the help they need as early as possible so that they can learn to manage it and achieve the happy, healthy adulthood that you dream for them.

My first experience with narcissism was similar to the way that many people first encounter this disorder—in an abusive partner. Like many women who find themselves in relationships with narcissistic men, it took me a very long time to realize that something was deeply wrong with the man that I had married, and by then it was far too late. His behavior toward me was almost certainly abusive, but the abuse was levelled in such a specific way that many people around me couldn't see it. As a successful author and athlete, I prided myself on my autonomy and power. It was humiliating for me to admit that I had not only become entrapped in an abusive relationship, but that even after divorce, I would have to co-parent my children with my abuser until I could convince a court of law that there was, indeed, something wrong with my ex-husband.

My determination to prove the destructive quality of my ex-husband's behavior eventually led me to the diagnosis that no one around us had been able to see through all the years of our marriage—narcissistic personality disorder. The more I learned about narcissism, *true* narcissism, the more fascinated I became. Five years later, I have gone on to professionally study not only narcissism but other personality disorders. With these years of clinical experience now behind me, my goal is to spread awareness of narcissistic personality disorder to as many people as I can possibly reach. It was only by learning the truth of this disorder that I was able to liberate myself from its negative influences. More importantly, it gave me insight into the life and the mind of the man that was partially raising my own children. After I gained an understanding of his disorder, I was able to coexist and co-parent with him in a way that was peaceful, stable, and even safe. Through knowledge, I was able to both heal from my ex-husband's abuse and even find a way to love and forgive him for his behavior. Had I known what I know now when I first met him, I would have avoided many years of pain, anger, and abuse.

More importantly, if my ex-husband's *parents* had known what I know now when he was a child, they may have been able to intervene at a critical point in his life, preventing him from growing into an abuser in the first place. I offer you this book so that you can intervene in your child's life in such a way. With knowledge, you can continue to be a loving parent to your child and get them the professional help they need before it's too late. With an understanding of the disorder and how to manage it, you can live together in peace, love, and understanding with narcissists of all ages and never fall prey to the infamously dark aspects of this disorder that so many have fallen victim to.

In this book, I offer you both personal insight and professional guidance. All of the information you find in this book will be supported by the latest science but will be relayed to you in ways that are easy for anyone to understand. It's my hope that this combination of wisdom and education will lead you and your child to the support that you need and thereby create a world that is safer and more loving for people of all personality types.

Chapter 1:

What Is a Narcissist?

With so much misinformation popularly available, it may be more useful to begin with what a narcissist *isn't*. Narcissists aren't simply people who are too full of themselves. The clinical diagnosis of narcissistic personality disorder is much more complex than that. Another popular myth is that narcissism is currently on the rise, especially in young people. However, there is no psychological evidence to support this.

In order to determine whether or not your child is a narcissist, you'll first need to have a clear understanding of what narcissism actually means from a clinical perspective. You may find that the strict psychological definition of narcissism is quite different from the popular cultural conception of the disorder. In order to recognize the warning signs of narcissism in your child, you'll need to know exactly what it is you're looking for.

Narcissism, in and of itself, is not a disorder—it's a personality trait. Like all personality traits, its manifestations are most accurately viewed as a spectrum, not a binary. Most people exhibit moderate levels of narcissism in their personality, with very few people showing extremely low or extremely high levels, both of which can be toxic. Narcissism in a person is traditionally measured using the Narcissistic Personality Inventory (or NPI), which was developed in 1979 by psychologists Robert Raskin and Calvin Hall. The test scores an individual on a scale of 0-40, with a score of between 10 and 20 considered "healthy." People with scores in the twenties are typically perceived as exceedingly charming by people who don't know them well and exceedingly vain by people who do. Narcissism at this level can certainly contribute to awkward or stressful interpersonal relationships, but it is still not a high enough score to constitute a personality disorder.

Though these traits may be annoying, someone who talks excessively about themself or never seems to experience self-doubt is not necessarily a narcissist. Excesses of self-esteem or insecurity actually have very little to do with a narcissism diagnosis. In fact, many narcissists are quite capable of recognizing that they are more self-centered than other people. At its core, narcissism is comprised of three main features: 1) hunger for appreciation or admiration, 2) desire to be the center of attention, and 3) expectations of special treatment reflecting perceived higher status. It's not surprising, then, that extremely high levels of narcissism can damage the quality of one's romantic, familial, or professional relationships. Even strong narcissistic tendencies can be damaging in people who are not aware of their disorder or the disorder of their loved one. People with high levels of narcissism tend to express feelings of antagonism, self-importance, and entitlement (*Narcissism,* n.d.).

Narcissists are characterized by a combination of a grandiose sense of self-importance, a lack of empathy for others, a need for excessive admiration, and a belief that one is unique or otherwise deserving of special treatment. If someone you know consistently exhibits all or most of these traits, it's very likely that they have a narcissistic personality.

Despite its prominent place in popular culture, narcissistic personality disorder is relatively rare, affecting less than one percent of the general population. It's typically diagnosed when a person's narcissistic traits begin to inhibit their ability to function normally in daily life. Most often, this dysfunction stems from the narcissist's characteristic lack of empathy. Antagonistic behavior in narcissists can also be fueled by their grandiosity or need for attention. People with narcissistic personality disorder see themselves as superior to others and so can become extremely rigid in the face of disagreement or questioning from others.

Strange though it may seem, if you suspect an adult of being a narcissist, the best way to find out is to simply ask them. It's another popular misconception that narcissists don't realize that they have a disorder. Psychologists have found that people who answer "yes" to the question "Are you a narcissist?" are significantly more likely to score higher on a narcissism evaluation than people who answer "no," even if the person has no preexisting diagnosis.

The reason that high levels of narcissism don't necessarily qualify as a disorder is because high levels of narcissism come with just as many benefits as they do weaknesses. Studies have found that people who score in the twenties on the NPI tend to exhibit increased levels of mental toughness and perform better than others in high-pressure situations. Children who score in this range have been found more likely to succeed in school. Adults with strong narcissistic tendencies also tend to perform better in the workplace due to higher levels of motivation and assertiveness. However, a clinical narcissist will exhibit these traits at a toxic level, always prioritizing getting ahead over getting along. Clinical narcissists are often uncollaborative, arrogant, and argumentative in the workplace. Because they are pathologically focused on "winning," they often take all the credit for team successes and retaliate against anyone they perceive to be disloyal (*Narcissism,* n.d.).

Maintaining a relationship of any kind with a narcissist can be distressing at best and outright abusive at worst. Because narcissists have a pathological need for admiration and control, they can be incredibly manipulative. Arguing with a narcissist rarely produces meaningful results. Instead, the most important way to protect yourself in a relationship with a narcissist is to establish firm boundaries. You cannot control your feelings toward someone else, but you *can* control how you express those feelings. Unfortunately, narcissistic partners or family members are often so far gone that you may have no choice but to emotionally distance yourself from them. Understanding what narcissism is and how to recognize it can also protect you from becoming trapped with a narcissistic boss and, of course, help you to better parent a narcissistic child.

When handling a narcissist, the two most important things you can do are acknowledge your frustration and appreciate where the other person's behaviors come from. The nature of your relationship with the narcissist in your life will change the way you handle them, as well. For example, the way that you manage a narcissistic boss is going to be slightly different from the way you manage a narcissistic child. The narcissistic boss is an unfortunately common problem because their inherent need for power and attention makes corporate management or even political leadership a natural place for them. However, true narcissists rarely last very long in positions of power because their primary focus is on self-promotion rather than advancing the goals of the organization.

Many people also find themselves in romantic partnerships with narcissists, and for understandable reasons. The narcissist's inherent desire for admiration can make them seem charming and charismatic in social situations. Narcissists often appear to have very high self-esteem. This often translates to a great deal of passion and charm in the early stages of a romantic relationship.

However, people experience problems when they realize that their narcissistic partner also has an inherent lack of empathy, making it extremely difficult for them to understand that other people have inner worlds. For the narcissist, their romantic partnerships are purely transactional. In exchange for positive attention and sexual satisfaction, the partner's primary responsibility is to boost the narcissist's ego and self-esteem. The ultimate goal for the narcissist is pleasure without commitment, and they will often lose interest in a relationship once there is a real expectation of intimacy from the other person (*Narcissism,* n.d.).

Unfortunately, it is almost impossible for people with narcissistic personality disorder to truly fall in love. Their need for absolute control often drives them to set very strict rules with romantic partners and can instigate abusive behaviors like isolating their partner from friends and family. Not every narcissist becomes a controlling abuser. Many narcissists find themselves serial daters, moving on from one short-term romantic partnership to the next. Many studies have found that narcissists exhibit higher levels of sociosexuality than other kinds of people, meaning they tend to have more hookups or casual dating experiences than committed relationships. While there is nothing inherently problematic about this approach to life, the narcissist's lack of empathy can often prevent them from being clear about their intentions or needs with their partner. They may present themselves as (falsely) wanting a committed relationship in order to attract a new partner or even pursue someone who is already in a monogamous relationship.

But remember that true narcissistic personality disorder is extremely rare. Someone who is periodically mean is very different from someone who inherently lacks empathy. All of us have our moments of selfishness, but a narcissist's entire worldview is unequivocally self-centered. It is almost impossible for them *not* to think selfishly, and this is the crux of the disorder, the root from which most of the narcissist's problematic behaviors stem.

Psychologists can subdivide narcissism into four basic types (more on this later). There are a few core traits that link all of the narcissistic personalities together. In addition to the NPI, psychologists use two different models for measuring an individual's personality traits thereby allowing them to determine which type (if any) of narcissism a person has.

The first of these models is called the Trifurcated Model of Narcissism, because it asserts that narcissism can be identified by examining three core traits: agentic extraversion, disagreeableness, and neuroticism. Agentic extroverts are people who are not only outgoing but authoritative and bold. The only trait that types one and two share is disagreeableness. The core trait shared by all four narcissistic types is interpersonal antagonism. This is a combination of manipulation, hostility, and entitlement that characterizes a narcissist's relationships.

The Narcissism Spectrum Model, on the other hand, is a very recent method of diagnosing narcissism, only discovered in 2017. This new model views narcissism on a spectrum from grandiose to vulnerable and insists that within that spectrum there is a great variety of severity and personality traits. In this model, the core of all narcissistic personalities is considered to be entitled self-importance. In other words, all types of narcissists believe that they and their needs are special (Lancer, 2020).

Measurements of Narcissism

The first and most widely-used tool to measure a narcissistic personality is a test called the NPI. Taking this assessment is commonly the first diagnostic step when someone is suspected of having narcissistic personality disorder (or NPD). This test is comprised of 40 items, each of which relates to a specific trait that theoretically corresponds to a narcissistic personality. Each question is designed to determine whether or not the individual being tested exhibits enough narcissistic traits to be diagnosed with NPD. These traits include feelings of superiority, willingness to exploit others, vanity, exhibitionism, authoritativeness, high self-sufficiency, and entitlement, among others. While this assessment is designed to evaluate narcissism, certain results can also indicate codependency or psychopathy (Foster, Shiverdecker, & Turner, 2016).

The NPI test is scored from 0 to 40, with results between 10 and 20 considered "healthy." Psychologists typically focus on the total score obtained by an individual. However, the test does not necessarily reflect the true variety of narcissistic traits or the many unique ways in which these traits can manifest themselves. The test is designed so that intrapersonal "healthy" narcissistic traits, such as leadership or superiority, are more pronounced in people with lower scores, while harmful traits, such as entitlement or being exploitative, are more pronounced in people with higher scores. In other words, the test does not simply determine whether you do or don't have NPD. It can also offer insight into the severity of an individual's narcissistic personality and which narcissistic traits they are more or less likely to exhibit.

If you're curious about how you (or someone else) may score on this exam, you don't have to pay for a professional. Psychcentral.com offers a free and accurate NPI evaluation under "quizzes," as does openpsychometrics.org, which can be found under "tests" (see the reference page for a link to this quiz). Remember that scores of between 10 and 20 are considered "healthy." Scores of 10 or below indicate codependency, scores in the twenties indicate strong narcissistic tendencies, scores in the thirties indicate narcissistic personality disorder, and a score of 40 indicates psychopathy. If you get any number that is not in the teens, you may want to consider reaching out to a professional (Psych Central Research Team, 2020).

Another surprisingly effective measurement of narcissism is called the Single Item Narcissism Scale, or SINS. This assessment presents the idea of a "narcissist" as someone who is egotistical, self-focused, and vain, and then asks the question: "To what extent do you agree with the statement 'I am a narcissist'?" The participant indicates their answer on a scale of 1 (not very true of me) to 7 (very true of me). This may seem like an absurdly simple way to measure a severe and rare disorder. A recent series of 11 experiments conducted by the Indiana University Lilly Family School of Philanthropy demonstrated that participant answers on this assessment are accurate predictors of NPD. These experiments sought to introduce the SINS to as many different kinds of people and in as many different contexts as possible. Some experiments surveyed undergraduate university students, for example, while others were conducted purely online. Less than 10 years after this study was published, the SINS has become a reputable diagnostic tool. In fact, results on the SINS are comparable with results on the NPI. One experiment in the study found that the different numbers on the SINS are roughly equivalent with the seven subscales of the NPI, which measure the seven narcissistic traits of vanity, exhibitionism, being exploitative, authority, superiority, self-sufficiency, and entitlement. Another found that people who take the SINS again after a period of 11 days are likely to get the exact same result. And yet another experiment found that people who scored themselves highly on the SINS were also much more likely to engage in risky sexual behaviors (*Just One Simple Question Can Identify Narcissistic People*, 2014).

The only important difference between these two evaluations is that the SINS is one simple question, while the NPI presents 40 different questions for a person to answer. Furthermore, this simple evaluation tells us that, contrary to popular belief, narcissists are relatively self-aware. People with NPD are typically proud of their narcissistic character traits. Unlike other disorders, narcissists typically don't view their atypical character traits as negative—in fact, feeling different from other people only feeds the idea that they are special or superior to others.

The ability to accurately diagnose narcissistic personalities has huge implications, not only for the narcissist but for all of the people affected by them. For example, narcissistic people have characteristically low empathy. Empathy is the primary motivator behind philanthropic behaviors like donating money to charitable organizations. Narcissists with the money to donate large sums to the well-being of others typically don't, which has potential implications for society as a whole. In this and many other ways, narcissism is both an individual and a social problem. People who already think they're great rarely work to improve themselves. People who only think about themselves are far less likely to help others.

Narcissism is a serious and rare disorder, so both the SINS and the NPI are typically used together to make an accurate diagnosis. The SINS is also limited, in the sense that it cannot indicate which type of narcissism someone has. This single-item test can be used as an early diagnostic tool, especially with people who may become fatigued or distracted by a long test. The average amount of time it takes to complete the SINS is 20 seconds, while it takes about 12 minutes to take the NPI. This can be a crucial time difference in studies with multiple tasks or when working with people who have a limited attention span, such as children (*Just One Simple Question Can Identify Narcissistic People,* 2016).

Like the NPI, a high SINS score isn't necessarily a bad thing, nor is it an automatic indicator of narcissistic personality disorder. People with high SINS scores also tend to be more extroverted and report more positive feelings about their lives. However, they also tend to report less agreeableness. The higher someone scores themselves on the SINS, the less likely they are to have healthy relationships with other people.

The biggest advantage of the SINS evaluation is that it helps professionals and laypeople to identify narcissists very easily. Someone who is willing to identify themselves as egotistical or self-concerned is very likely to have other psychological or personality problems. There's no need to continue on to a more thorough assessment like the NPI if someone scores very low on the SINS.

But short of taking an official evaluation, what are the common traits of a narcissist? There are a few key traits to watch for, especially when more than two or three seem to appear in the same person. This list of traits was originally compiled by Otto Kernberg, one of the leading psychoanalysts of the 20th century (Stines, 2019):

- *Frequent lies and exaggerations.* Narcissists often attempt to make themselves seem special or superior to others by showing off, bragging, taking undeserved credit, or using other forms of self-aggrandizement. Worse, narcissists have a tendency to bolster their own self-image by putting others down. They often seek to make others feel inferior through false accusations or constant criticism. They are adept at distorting the facts, willing to tell deliberate lies if those lies will further their own agenda. No matter what, the ultimate goal of any narcissistic lie or exaggeration is to boost their surprisingly fragile sense of self-worth (Ni, 2017).

- *Need for constant adulation and attention.* The primary source of satisfaction in a narcissist's life is attention from other people. This attention can be positive or negative, as long as it involves a flow of emotional energy from the other person to the narcissist.

- *Rarely admit flaws.* Narcissists have very thin skin and can become extremely aggressive in response to criticism. When challenged, they regress to a fight or flight response. More extroverted kinds of narcissists tend to respond to criticism with aggressive behaviors like temper tantrums, excuses, denial, blame, and hypersensitivity, while more introverted types tend to respond with passive-aggressive behaviors like disappearing, avoidance, silent treatment, sulking, or resentment. Rather than owning up to their deceptions, narcissists will cling ever tighter to their false accusations. Narcissists tend to view relationships as competitive rather than collaborative. As such, they respond strongly to criticism because they view it as a personal attack (Ni, 2017).

- *False image projection.* Narcissists project a false, idealized image of themselves to the world in order to hide their inner insecurities. They try to impress others by focusing on external markers of success. The false identity built by narcissists can be physical, romantic, sexual, social, religious, financial, material, professional, academic, cultural, or a combination (Ni, 2017). No matter what, the purpose of the false image is to send the message "I'm better than you!" They see themselves as the dominant presence in personal or professional relationships. Narcissists often believe themselves to be all-powerful or superhumanly strong. They can bolster their own egos and even take pride in marginalizing those they perceive to be weaker than they are. This can give their interpersonal relationships an edge of cruelty (sometimes more than an edge). Narcissists want other people to worship them, and the construction of a false image is part of satisfying that need. Their external facades are built to replace their real and insecure selves (Ni, 2017).

- *Rule breaking and boundary violations.* Narcissists presume entitlement and therefore take a narrow, egocentric view of other people. This can sometimes lead them to oppress or even dehumanize the people around them.
- *Emotional invalidation and coercion.* Narcissists typically and frequently invalidate the thoughts, feelings, and priorities of those around them. While all people do this occasionally, narcissists show little or no remorse when they realize their behavior has caused someone else pain.
- *Manipulation.* Simply put, manipulation is the tendency to make decisions for others based on one's own agenda. Narcissists, in particular, often use guilt, blame, and victimhood as manipulative tools. It can be easy for them to fool others because their extreme confidence makes them sound like experts in whatever they're talking about. They can also be quite convincing when arguing their point, even if that point is nonsensical or has negative implications if the other person agrees. Gaslighting is a particularly insidious manipulative tool that narcissists use frequently. Gaslighting is technically a form of brainwashing that causes paralyzing feelings of self-doubt in the victim. In the long-term, gaslighting can cause a victim to lose their sense

of perception and identity. This is so common, in fact, that multiple studies have been done on narcissistic gaslighting, especially in romantic relationships. That being said, not everyone who gaslights is a narcissist, and not every narcissist employs gaslighting. But the chronic use of this manipulation technique is a strong indicator of NPD (Ni, 2017).

- *Frequent lying.* Everyone lies sometimes. Narcissists are just as likely to lie as they are to tell the truth.
- *Delusional or fantasy thinking.* Narcissists typically engage in delusions when they can't get enough attention from other people, including self-aggrandizement fantasies or the idealization of a new romantic partner. Despite their appearance of high self-esteem, narcissism ultimately begins when someone buries their ability to honestly express themself. The alternate persona that they create as a result is one of grandiosity and superiority.
- *Chronic boredom.* Narcissists frequently complain of boredom or dissatisfaction with their lives, a state that they typically expect those around them to fix.
- *High degree of self-reference in conversations.* Narcissists think about everything in reference to themselves. As such, people in close

relationships often find themselves becoming "other-referenced," or making decisions based on how they think the narcissist will react, rather than what is best for themselves.

- *No disordered appearance.* The first impression most narcissists make is one of warmth, friendliness, and social affability. The more intelligent the narcissist, the better they are with people—at least at first.
- *High sense of self-importance.* The crucial narcissistic contradiction is that this high sense of self-worth must be reinforced with constant praise from other people. This is the essential difference between narcissism and true self-confidence. Truly confident people don't need a constant stream of validation from others.
- *Shallow emotions.* Narcissists are unable to tolerate intense negative feelings like sadness or guilt. They also become extremely agitated by any strong displays of emotion in other people.
- *No care for the feelings of others.* Narcissists see other people as obsessions and so have very little concern for how other people feel. The only feelings that are important to a narcissist are their own.
- *Frequent feelings of envy.* Narcissists are often extremely jealous or resentful of other people.

This stems from the deep-seated belief that they deserve what other people have.

- *Extreme feelings of entitlement.* Narcissists tend to take problems and challenges in life personally. They respond to life's difficulties with anger, resentment, and contempt. They believe that if they don't get their way, something is wrong.
- *Idolization and deprecation.* Narcissists interact with people in one of two ways. They idolize those who give them the attention they crave and deprecate those who don't.
- *Rapid emotional expression.* Narcissists can move very quickly from anger to calm and back again. Strong emotions can come on very suddenly and can vanish easily as fast.
- *Extreme independence.* Narcissists are extremely self-sufficient, to the point that they sometimes appear detached or aloof from other people.
- *Extremely unpredictable.* Their emotional instability makes narcissists very difficult to predict.
- *Extreme defensiveness.* Projective identification, apparent omnipotence, idealization of the self or others, denial, rage attacks, yelling, blame, projection, and gaslighting are all weapons commonly used by narcissists when they feel criticized or challenged.

- *Extreme selfishness and self-centeredness.* Narcissists are only happy when their needs are being met 100% of the time, regardless of what that might mean for the people around them.

If you suspect you are in some kind of relationship with a narcissist, these are the traits to watch for. While all of us display these traits at low points in our lives, narcissists display them all the time. They have no capacity to grow beyond these behaviors and so have no capacity to care for the emotional well-being of the people around them (Stines, 2019).

The Narcissism Spectrum

Cultural usage of the word "narcissist" has been on the rise over the past 10 years. Often, however, the word is used as an insult. Most people don't want to be known as a narcissist or publicly called out when they engage in narcissistic behavior. The underlying needs of the narcissist, however, are actually quite universal. Every human needs to be praised by parents or caregivers during childhood, and narcissists are typically adults that didn't get enough of this kind of validation early in life (Soeiro, 2019).

In 1914, Sigmund Freud proposed that all human infants are narcissists, in the sense that their brains simply aren't capable of understanding that other people are separate, autonomous entities. This, he asserted, was a perfectly normal and healthy part of human development. Narcissists, however, are people who manage to grow into adulthood without fully leaving this stage of development behind them. Karen Horney, one of Freud's successors, expanded this research, positing that children who received excessive amounts of attention or neglect would grow into narcissistic adults obsessed with getting validation from other people. Later in the 20th century, Otto Kernberg would define the narcissistic personality as a kind of internal defense mechanism, a false front to protect someone from their insecurities. He argued that the narcissist's grandiose persona was a way for them to validate themselves when they weren't getting enough attention from other people. The narcissistic persona, then, is a kind of elaborate mask constructed to hide a very fragile self-esteem (Narcissist Abuse Support, 2019).

Today we understand that narcissism is not a unitary condition. Like many other disorders, it exists on a spectrum. Tests like the NPI have allowed psychologists to see the many different shades and nuances from narcissism, on a scale from normal to pathological. The lowest end of the spectrum (10 or lower on the NPI) is codependency. This is not a personality disorder but a behavioral one. People who are codependent have a cripplingly low sense of self-worth and so are unable to find happiness without being in some kind of relationship. Even though, codependents will often sacrifice their entire lives to the relationship, drawing their sense of identity from the relationship and simultaneously entangling their partner to ensure they never leave. Perhaps unsurprisingly, these kinds of people often find themselves in relationships with people who have narcissistic personality disorder.

In some ways, codependency can be seen as the complete lack of narcissism, which is why a "healthy" score on the NPI is not necessarily the lowest. We all need a little bit of narcissism in order to feel happy and function normally in the world. Without it, we find ourselves utterly powerless in our relationships and entirely without autonomy over our lives.

The next shade of narcissism is often referred to as "subclinical" narcissism (20-29 on the NPI). These people display strong narcissistic traits but don't display those traits with enough severity or intensity to be diagnosed with full-blown narcissistic personality disorder. The reason for this is that subclinical narcissists may have trouble finding healthy or happy relationships, but in other ways, they benefit from their narcissistic traits. Studies have linked subclinical narcissism with increased mental toughness, better resilience in high-pressure situations, and increased productivity in the workplace. A narcissist's heightened sense of self can make them more motivated and assertive than others. And many studies have found that narcissists are much less likely to experience depression than other people (*Narcissism,* n.d.).

Within subclinical and clinical narcissism, we find four distinct narcissistic types, which also exist on a scale from domineering and extroverted to neurotic and introverted. Each type of narcissist will require a different approach in order for you to have a happy and healthy relationship with them. All four types are invested in making those around them feel insecure in order to assure their social status. Each type will use different tactics to achieve that goal. As such, it's important to not only identify whether or not someone is a narcissist, but which type of narcissist they are.

Type One - The Grandiose Narcissist

It would be fair to call this the "classic" narcissist, as this is the first type of narcissism recognized by psychology and is the type that most literature on "narcissism" is really discussing. These people are boastful and often find themselves in the limelight as public figures.

Grandiose narcissists are typically charming but attention-seeking extroverts. Common traits include self-absorption, entitlement, and callousness. Because they are inherently unempathetic, many become physically abusive. Grandiose narcissists are often arrogant, thinking extremely highly of themselves while having a very low opinion of others.

Grandiose narcissists rarely recognize that they have a disorder because their extroversion and high self-esteem often lead to great satisfaction with their lives. Grandiose narcissism is an externalized disorder because they outwardly seek acclaim and attention. This remains true (and becomes particularly problematic) in romantic relationships. Many grandiose narcissists do manage to maintain ongoing partnerships by seducing others with their charisma and boldness (Lancer, 2020).

Subclinical type ones are exhibitionistic, self-absorbed, and continuously seeking ways to stay in the limelight. They may be authoritarian and aggressive but not enough to be considered abusive. Those with NPD, however, are also entitled, callous, and often exploitative. This is the most common type of NPD, but it can be the most difficult to diagnose, as most type ones report high self-esteem and satisfaction with their lives, even if they know that their actions are causing others pain.

Type Two - The Vulnerable Narcissist

This type is often referred to as the "covert" or "closet" narcissist. People with this type of narcissism are just as self-absorbed as those with type one, but they have a deep, pathological fear of criticism. Both type one and type two narcissists lack personal autonomy and experience imposter syndrome in positions of power. The vulnerable narcissist experiences these things with much greater intensity.

While grandiose narcissists often feel confident and self-satisfied, vulnerable narcissists feel insecure and unhappy. These people experience a great deal of distress, anxiety, and guilt throughout their lives. They swing between having an irrationally positive and an irrationally negative view of themselves, but either way, their self-image is greatly removed from reality. Their general negativity makes it almost impossible for them to self-reflect or engage in any kind of personal growth. Their grandiose self-image requires a great deal of reinforcement, and they can become extremely defensive when they believe they're being criticized.

Vulnerable narcissism is an introverted personality type. These types of people experience relationships from a threat-oriented and inherently distrustful position. Most of them have avoidant or anxious attachment styles. They tend to unleash a lot of blame and resentment on anyone who manages to get too close. For this reason, empathetic codependents often find themselves in relationships with vulnerable narcissists.

Subclinical type twos tend to shy away from the limelight because their fear of criticism causes them so much distress. They may experience high levels of anxiety and guilt, but these same feelings are what often cause them to seek professional help. Those with NPD, however, also experience high levels of depression, hypersensitivity, and shame. These people become extremely defensive whenever they perceive themselves to be criticized as their self-worth is entirely dependent on positive reinforcement from other people (Lancer, 2020).

Type Three - The Communal Narcissist

This type of narcissist is perhaps the most difficult to identify. These kinds of narcissists actively value warmth and agreeableness. They see themselves as the most trustworthy and supportive person in any social setting. This makes them outgoing, like the grandiose narcissist. Instead of proving that they are the smartest or the most powerful person in the room, the communal narcissist is obsessed with proving that they are the most giving and helpful. Though the communal narcissist often appears selfless, the reality is that this image of friendliness and kindness is what gives them power over others. In this way, they share the same goals of grandiosity and esteem as type one narcissists—they just employ a very different method of achieving them. If their hypocrisy is discovered, they can become just as defensive or abusive as the other narcissistic types.

Subclinical type threes see themselves as the most trustworthy and supportive person in the room. They constantly try to prove this through acts of friendliness and kindness, which rarely causes problems in relationships that aren't close or intimate. Those with NPD, however, become obsessed with proving to others that they are the most giving and helpful, with the same intensity that type ones experience when trying to prove themselves the most powerful. This obsession with proving themselves to be the best causes similar problems to type ones. Their ultimate goals are the achievement of grandiosity, esteem, entitlement, and power—they just go about achieving those goals in a very different way.

Type Four - The Malignant Narcissist

This is the rarest type of narcissism. Malignant narcissists share many of their basic personality traits with grandiose narcissists, but they add to the mix extremes of paranoia and immorality. These kinds of narcissists find extreme pleasure in creating chaos. Not all of them are grandiose or extroverted, but all malignant narcissists are neurotic and obsessed with taking other people down.

Even subclinical type fours are cruel, aggressive, and paranoid. They can show themselves to be immoral and sadistic, even at a young age. These NPD types take these qualities to an extreme level, finding pleasure in creating chaos and taking other people down. Type fours typically score very high on the NPI (28-30 and 38-40), and those who score a perfect 40 are not actually narcissists at all. They have a different, but related, personality disorder—psychopathy.

When trying to identify the type of narcissist you're dealing with, it's important to remember that grandiose narcissists often swing between states of extreme grandiosity and extreme vulnerability. Their vulnerability often shows when their success has been thwarted or their self-concept has been challenged. In general, the more grandiose a narcissist's personality, the more unstable their emotions are. Vulnerable narcissists, on the other hand, almost never exhibit grandiosity.

Narcissistic personality disorder is the most intense expression of narcissism. One of many personality disorders, it is typically suspected when a person's narcissistic traits begin to disrupt their ability to function in relationships, work, or school. Often, it's the narcissist's lack of empathy that first triggers problems in personal relationships. Narcissists can become dangerously unhappy when they don't receive the special favors they believe they're owed. They often find their relationships unfulfilling, and others increasingly dislike being around them (*Narcissistic Personality Disorder - Symptoms and Causes,* 2017).

Unfortunately, the more severe a person's narcissism, the more resistant they can be to treatment. It's in the nature of the disorder for the narcissist to believe that they are perfect, even special. If they do agree to seek treatment, it's often for depression or substance abuse. A diagnosis of a personality disorder can be extremely difficult for people with NPD to accept. If you recognize the signs and symptoms of narcissistic personality disorder in yourself or your loved ones, it's important to find professional help right away. Though it is a severe disorder, proper management of the symptoms can make life far more rewarding for both the narcissist and the people around them. While many people display characteristics of subclinical narcissism, narcissistic personality disorder itself is relatively rare, affecting less than 6% of the general population (Johnson, 2017). Treatment for the disorder typically consists of talk therapy.

Understanding narcissism as a spectrum is a relatively new approach to recognizing and treating the disorder, developed as recently as 2017. However, this new look at the disorder has offered psychologists and laypeople alike a much more accurate view of the disorder, giving everyone the ability to see the many ways that narcissism can manifest in a person's psyche. The four different types of narcissism are essentially different narcissistic traits manifesting themselves in more or less intense ways. The more grandiose types (one and three) have less vulnerability in their personalities, while the more neurotic types (two and four) have more vulnerability and therefore less grandiosity.

These four types of narcissism, then, exist on a sliding scale of traits, from extroverted to introverted, from domineering to neurotic. The more extroverted types are more grandiose. These types tend to score lower on the NPI and also tend to feel and function better than the neurotic types. However, no matter how socially engaging they may be, their antagonism will eventually come out and destroy their intimate relationships.

The more vulnerable types, on the other hand, tend to score higher on the NPI and need professional help in dealing with their perceptions and moods. Because their emotions are so intense, they have been often misdiagnosed with borderline personality disorder in the past, especially type twos. These types can benefit greatly from dialectical behavior therapy, which can help them to manage their antagonism.

Those with clinical narcissism can be further divided into two subtypes—"prosocial" or "antisocial." Those who are prosocial have much less antagonism and much more self-absorption than those who are antisocial, where these traits are flipped. The current cultural perception of the narcissist as a selfish schemer who will gladly misuse relationships for their own benefit has much more to do with the antisocial type than with the prosocial. Antisocial narcissists can, indeed, be extremely difficult and self-centered people. Prosocial narcissists crave positive attention. They make it their mission to do as many good deeds as possible—they just perform these deeds where they're sure others will notice. The motivation behind these good deeds is the same thing that drives all narcissists in one way or another—validation.

Prosocial narcissists can be more difficult to spot because most of the time, they're a great deal of fun. They want to be liked, but they take that want to an extreme level. They are driven by the deep-seated need to be known and appreciated by everyone around them. Unlike their antisocial counterparts, they do have low levels of empathy, which they use to determine what's going to most please the people around them.

In general, prosocial narcissists tend to be types one and three, while antisocial tend to be types two and four. Type fours, in particular, frequently lash out at other people in order to bolster their own self-worth. This type was first discovered in the 1980s, before which it was often misdiagnosed as antisocial personality disorder. Subclinical type fours can manage to have long-term relationships, but their behavior is incredibly unstable. They are considered a neurotic type because they do a great deal of inner work to protect their grandiose self-concept. Antisocial narcissists of all types lie frequently and become quite angry when they get caught. Antisocial narcissists see all social interactions as a kind of contest, one that they are determined to win (Soeiro, 2019).

Type twos can also be considered an antisocial type. Just like the other types, twos believe that they are superior to other people, but they are the best at hiding those feelings. Vulnerable narcissists are extremely self-absorbed and do a great deal of inner work to maintain their inflated sense of self. Inflated self-image makes them feel like they deserve more attention than they get, which, in turn, makes them view themselves as chronically victimized. Twos are the only type of narcissist that are vulnerable to depression. Their great depth of emotion, however, is often mistaken for hypersensitivity.

By viewing narcissism as a spectrum, we are able to see the core traits of antagonism, self-importance, and entitlement as they manifest themselves in varying degrees of intensity. This new spectrum model has caused an explosion of research in the past few years, helping psychologists to make huge strides in both better understanding narcissism and better distinguishing it from other personality disorders like sociopathy or borderline (Lancer, 2020).

The ability to see narcissism as a spectrum is also valuable for those in relationships with a narcissist. Maintaining a healthy relationship with a narcissist can be an exhausting task. Rather than getting their needs met, those who are close to narcissists often feel undermined and emotionally drained. Instead of becoming more intimate, they find themselves struggling for the narcissist's positive attention and walking on eggshells to avoid offending them. Loved ones are constantly disappointed when the narcissist, time and again, prioritizes themself over everyone else. If you recognize any of these features in someone close to you, don't waste any more energy trying to please or change the narcissistic person in your life. Instead, recognize them for who they are. Take note of their narcissistic traits and how they manifest in different settings. The more familiar you are with the full range of the narcissism spectrum, the better you will be at setting healthy boundaries and take steps to protect your own self-worth. Individual psychotherapy can often be valuable and necessary for both the narcissist and their loved ones.

Chapter 2:

Inside the Narcissistic

Mind

Now that you know the basics of narcissism, it's time to take a closer look at the mind of a narcissist. What motivates them? What makes them tick?

If your child is truly narcissistic, you won't be able to help them if you can't understand the motivations behind their behaviors. For example, a typical child will throw a tantrum as a way to assert their autonomy or signal to their parents that something is wrong. A narcissistic child may throw a tantrum as a ploy for attention or to force you to do as they say. To effectively handle them, you'll need to have a clear understanding of what motivations lie beneath your child's more destructive behaviors.

When thinking about the narcissistic mind, the most important question to answer is: Do narcissists *know* they're narcissists?

Traditionally, it's been assumed that narcissists are not self-aware. As introduced in Chapter 1, a recent diagnostic tool called the SINS exam has found that, when asked the question "Are you a narcissist?" most people are able to answer with relative honesty, including narcissists themselves. The success of this new tool has led psychologists to believe that, in the past, narcissists have denied their condition because it's been presented to them as a diagnosis, which they take as an insult. But when the condition is presented to them in neutral terms, they are able to own up to their narcissistic traits, which they believe to be benefits, not flaws, in their character.

However, diagnostic tools only provide us with the clinical guidelines needed to *diagnose* someone with narcissism. This gives mental health professionals a degree of uniformity and clarity when making diagnostic decisions, but diagnostic criteria do not necessarily provide insight into a narcissist's true character or inner nature.

There are a few insights that we can gain from the diagnostic criteria listed in the DSM-5. Short for the Diagnostic and Statistical Manual of Mental Disorders, the DSM-5 is a standardized, official listing of every psychological disorder that's officially recognized by licensed mental health providers in the United States. According to this official listing, to qualify for NPD, a person must exhibit all three of these personality traits since early adulthood:

- a never-ending need for attention.
- a grandiose self-image, whether that image is based in real achievements or is purely

imagined. This is expressed through constant exaggeration of abilities, accomplishments, and/or talents.

- a noticeable lack of empathy.

In addition to these three traits, the person must also exhibit at least five of the following traits (*Narcissistic personality disorder - Symptoms and Causes*, 2017):

- having an exaggerated sense of self-importance
- exaggerating achievements or talents
- expecting to be recognized as superior without the achievements to earn such respect
- being preoccupied with fantasies of unlimited success, power, brilliance, beauty, or the perfect romantic partner
- believing that they are special and can only be understood by or associate with other special people
- monopolizing conversations and belittling others
- expecting special favors and unquestioning compliance from others
- requiring excessive admiration
- having a sense of entitlement, requiring constant, excessive admiration
- selfishly taking advantage of others to fulfill their own agenda

- lacking empathy or an inability to recognize the needs and feelings of others
- having frequent feelings of envy or believing that others are envious of them
- showing arrogant, haughty, patronizing, conceited, or boastful behaviors
- insisting on having the best of everything, such as the best office or the most expensive car

In addition to these traits, people with NPD can also:

- become extremely impatient when they don't receive special treatment
- have significant problems maintaining interpersonal relationships
- react with rage or contempt to anything they perceive to be a criticism
- have difficulty regulating their emotions
- have difficulty managing stress
- feel extremely depressed when they fall short of perfection
- harbor secret feelings of intense insecurity and shame

These criteria tell us what to look for and how to spot NPD. What they don't tell us is how such a person might think or feel in their day-to-day lives. The reality is that very few people actually meet these criteria. However, that does not take into account the number of romantic partners, spouses, parents, and other kinds of people who have been negatively affected by their relationships with these people. It's also true that those who exhibit strong narcissistic traits can still engage with the same problematic behaviors and motivations as those with an outright diagnosis. In other words, you don't necessarily need a diagnosis of NPD to be a narcissist (Bergeron, 2019).

In recent years, the word "narcissist" has become an increasingly popular insult hurled at those we perceive to be self-centered or selfish. These traits, though, have very little to do with the realities of narcissism. Worse, the popular prevalence of the word can distort the common conception of what a narcissist is, making it harder for both narcissists and their loved ones to get the help they need. Remember that narcissism is a spectrum and that healthy individuals exhibit narcissist traits, too.

Narcissists have a way of appearing very engaging and charming in social situations. Their motivations are often very different from what you might expect them to be. Narcissists live by their own internal code, based on the core values of getting attention and preserving self-image. This code is often at the root of the narcissist's problematic or harmful behaviors, including their incessant boasts, put-downs, and general volatility. This code is instinctive and often entirely unconscious on the narcissist's part. Understanding it can make the narcissist in your life feel less unpredictable and significantly more manageable.

Image is everything. Looking good is vitally important to all narcissists. They will either viciously attack or attempt to conceal anything that makes them look bad. This is why they can react in extreme ways if they feel slighted or insulted. Almost all of their problematic behaviors, including shaming, guilting, and attacking, are triggered when their self-image is threatened. Gaslighting is a masterful way for them to distract others from their flaws or shift the responsibility for their behavior onto someone else.

Narcissists assume that everyone around them is absolutely entranced by and in awe of them. When they feel ignored or when other people don't cater specifically to their needs, this idealized sense of self is threatened. This triggers the deep-seated fear that maybe they are not as beautiful or superior as they believe themselves to be. Narcissists have a highly inflated sense of self, but that self-image is extremely fragile. Preserving their grandiose self-image in the eyes of others is important, but they also go to great lengths to prove it to themselves. Preservation of their ego structure is vital to their well-being. Without it, they experience a catastrophic crisis of identity. This is what makes their sense of self-awareness so limited. This is also why narcissists rarely admit that they were wrong or apologize for anything. They believe that apologizing is a sign of weakness rather than respect. They fear that if they admit to being wrong about one thing, the other person will start to question what else they may be wrong about. If you do manage to get an apology out of a narcissist, it's usually a sarcastic one (Neuharth, 2019).

Attention is essential. Attention is fundamental to a narcissist's psychology. When narcissists feel listened to or admired, this takes them to the peak of their confidence and power. When attention from others is scarce, however, they experience a kind of withdrawal, becoming irritable or even depressed. Like an addict that has run through their supply, the narcissist will do whatever it takes to get the attention they need to thrive.

The narcissist's self-image is built entirely around what other people think of them and has nothing to do with who they actually are. As such, it's extremely painful for them to be alone. Attention from others provides the proof they need that they are special and worthy of love. The children and partners of narcissists are perhaps the best witnesses to just how much attention can make a narcissist blossom.

Honesty is optional. For most people, being honest is more important than being right. For the narcissist, it's the opposite. Narcissists value expediency far more than they value authenticity.

This makes them adept liars. Narcissists are infamous for how convincing they can be in their arguments. This is because their innate belief in their own "rightness" lends the lie an air of truth—they almost believe themselves. To them, their opinion about the truth is just as valid as any "objective" truth. They believe that the truth is malleable. Whatever they think or feel in the moment is what is "honest," regardless of how that relates to the current reality of the situation. Speaking with absolute certainty isn't difficult for narcissists because they always feel stronger and better than the person they're talking to. If the other person believes them, they feel that much more validated.

Danger is everywhere. Though it often appears to be the opposite, narcissists carry within them a great deal of fear. Their image of confidence is just an image. They rarely show it, but inside, they believe that others are primarily motivated to humiliate or beat them in social situations. Because they are inherently suspicious of other people's motivations, they rarely pursue intimate relationships and rarely communicate openly with others. As such, what relationships they do have tend to become parasitic, with the flow of intimacy and trust moving in one direction only (Neuharth, 2019).

Most people share a great deal about themselves with others. Narcissists never ask for help and never allow themselves to show any vulnerability. They never let themselves express negative emotions like sadness or loneliness. Expressing our true emotions is the primary way that we connect with others. Because narcissists never do this, they find themselves viewing all social interactions through the lens of conflict. Challenging and dominating is the only way they know how to interact with other people.

Consistency is overrated. A narcissist's behaviors are primarily governed by emotions and impulses. As such, they rarely pause to consider the long-term consequences of their actions. The narcissist's internal reality is continually shifting in an attempt to preserve their grandiose sense of self. Their attitudes, beliefs, and opinions can change day by day, or even hour by hour. Perhaps surprisingly, narcissists are fully self-aware of their emotional volatility, but it's something they often perceive as a strength, as it forces the people around them to constantly guess what the narcissist will do next.

Introspection is unnecessary. Contrary to popular belief, narcissists are capable of introspection—they just choose not to engage with it. They don't want to know why they do what they do, and they certainly aren't interested in making any changes. They aren't concerned with cultivating themselves; they are concerned with cultivating their image. Narcissists fear self-reflection because it might expose flaws or personal shame. Many also worry that engaging in self-reflection might distract or otherwise prevent them from getting what they want. It's this complete lack of introspection that makes it very difficult for narcissists to take responsibility for their dysfunctional behaviors. Unfortunately, it's this lack of personal accountability that also makes it so difficult for them to change.

Ironically, the only people a narcissist truly respects are people they believe to be just as perfect and special as they are. The only people they will pursue intimate relationships with are people that they have somehow idealized. Just as they cannot face themselves for who they truly are, they also cannot take a balanced or objective view of other people.

Winning is mandatory. Narcissists have what psychologists call an "ego-syntonic" mindset. This means that they never think they are responsible for any problems their behavior may cause. When something goes wrong, they genuinely believe that others are at fault, no matter how clear it is to the contrary. This is because they cannot understand that the needs of others are as important as their own needs (Bergeron, 2019).

One of the most problematic features of the narcissistic personality is their lack of empathy. This prevents them from being able to see a situation from someone else's point of view. The narcissist's entire life is centered around winning. They will sacrifice anything and everyone in order to be the best. Worse, narcissists also expect that those around them will do what's best for *them* and have no awareness or empathy for what that might cost the other person. Narcissists don't believe in win-wins because these situations rob them of their advantage. Instead, narcissists will turn any and every interaction into a game of credit and blame.

However, their lack of empathy or interest in other people's feelings means that they rarely notice when they've hurt or offended someone. If they do notice, however, they are unlikely to care. Some narcissists even come to enjoy upsetting other people. They thrive off the negative attention and power it gives them (Neuharth, 2019).

Narcissists only view other people in terms of what those people can provide for them. In order for them to value someone, that "special" someone is required to support the narcissist's view of themselves as perfect and flawless. Anyone who challenges that view is viciously rejected. Often, they feel extremely hurt and betrayed by family members, friends, or romantic partners who dare to suggest they may be less than perfect. On the flip side, those who enter into romantic relationships with narcissists often feel lavished with affection and attention at first, only to have that affection violently withdrawn at the slightest provocation.

All of this paints a relatively dark picture of what it's like to live with a narcissist or to live with the disorder yourself. Understanding what motivates a narcissist can give us the compassion we need to cope with their behaviors in a safe and healthy way. It can also help us to better understand our own narcissistic wounds. The lowest end of the narcissistic spectrum (those who score less than a 10 on the NPI) have another self-esteem related condition called codependency. Narcissists and codependents almost always end up in romantic partnerships with each other. Codependents have almost no sense of self-worth and so are ready and willing to devote their entire lives to the narcissist, who subsequently thrives off the unending stream of attention. The codependent has no ability to challenge the narcissist's superiority, which confirms the narcissist's feelings of power and unlimited authority. However, this kind of relationship also makes the narcissist dependent on their codependent partner. They become addicted to the attention administered by the codependent, attention that they cannot get from anyone else in their lives. The more the codependent's identity dissolves into the narcissist's ego, the less able the narcissist is to preserve that ego without support from the codependent (Bergeron, 2019).

Ultimately, most of what narcissists do and say is motivated by a need to protect their extremely fragile self-esteem. What can be most hurtful for loved ones is coming to terms with the fact that the narcissist in your life can never show you compassion in return. When coping with narcissists, it's critical to remember that they are extremely manipulative. Always think critically about anything a narcissist has said to you, and never take anything at face value. Instead, ask yourself the following questions whenever you find yourself feeling pressured, bullied, or intimidated:

- What is the cost of tolerating this behavior? What are the benefits?
- What is the cost of resisting this behavior? What are the benefits?

Remember that it is always OK for you to do what's good for *you*.

Approaches and Insights to Narcissistic Motivations

Narcissistic people across the spectrum are self-absorbed and grandiose, so much so that it damages their personal relationships. Even those who don't meet all the diagnostic criteria for NPD can still frustrate and irritate the people close to them. The most noticeable narcissistic trait is their need for constant attention. Boasting about their accomplishments, posting self-inflating pictures of themself on social media, or claiming connections with powerful people are all behaviors that stand out, especially when they're a constant feature of someone's communication style. The common mistake people make is that narcissists do these things because they want other people to like them.

Status vs. Affiliation

Throughout their lives, most people try to balance their desire to be liked with their desire to be respected. In psychology, these desires are commonly referred to as the desire for *status* (respect) and *affiliation* (being liked). Maintaining this balance is what helps us to build close connections with other people without losing our own autonomy. But as we all know, this is far easier said than done. Often, these two desires come into conflict with one another (Zeigler-Hill, 2019). For example, a manager who remains cold and professional in the workplace may earn the respect of their employees but may not be liked by them very much. By contrast, a manager who is constantly laughing and joking with the employees may be liked by all, but their authority as a manager may not be respected.

In narcissists, however, these desires are out of balance all the time. Their desire to be respected far outweighs their desire to be liked. This causes them to place too much importance on social status and not enough on building positive relationships. Whenever they experience a conflict, they always choose to fulfil their desire for status. Viewing narcissists in this way can offer a great deal of insight into their behaviors. When seen in this light, obnoxious and socially inappropriate behaviors like bragging about their accomplishments or flaunting their wealth begin to make more sense.

In recent years, there has been a significant amount of research done on the narcissistic obsession with status vs. affiliation. One of the necessary diagnostic requirements for NPD is the excessive need for admiration, which is what causes narcissists to exhibit their positive qualities and fuels their high assertiveness. Another quality related to this internal conflict is called *narcissistic rivalry*. This is what happens when narcissists believe that they are not getting the attention or being valued by others as much as they deserve. In a recent study, a group of participants was asked to rate the importance of a list of motivations in their lives, including status, affiliation, self-protection, finding a romantic partner, keeping their current romantic partner, caring for their family, and caring for their physical health. The study found narcissistic participants almost always ranked "status" as their most important motivator. Another study that tracked participants' emotional reactions to daily experiences found that narcissistic participants were far more sensitive to events involving status than to events concerning affiliation. Specifically, days on which they felt respected or admired by others corresponded with a significant increase in general feelings of well-being. These feelings of well-being did not seem to be triggered by any other events in the participants' lives, even events that could be objectively seen as positive (Zeigler-Hill, 2019).

The desire for status also plays a strong role for narcissists in romantic relationships. The extent to which narcissists are satisfied in their romantic partnerships is almost entirely dependent on how much they believe their partner respects them. This is in contrast to most people, who tend to place relatively equal importance on how much their partner both respects and likes them.

The narcissist's desire for status is so intense that, in many ways, it can be viewed as the narcissist's central motivation. It's the thing around which they structure their entire lives and may be the primary way in which they communicate their value and worthiness to those around them.

The Inner Critic

Narcissists are very easy to recognize but much more difficult to understand. The motivations behind their behavior can be baffling because they are very different from the motivations experienced by most other people. Their inflated sense of self can obscure the insecurities that not only hide beneath it but arguably give it life. Understanding a narcissist's inner voice is another way to understand why they do what they do.

Remember, the three critical criteria for an NPD diagnosis are grandiosity, excessive need for admiration, and a lack of empathy. These three traits do not manifest themselves exactly the same way in every narcissist. Grandiose narcissists may appear arrogant and entitled. Vulnerable narcissists, on the other hand, may appear deeply resentful and require constant reassurance from others. The underlying commonality between these two seemingly different personalities is the excessive need to compare themselves with others. Grandiose narcissists may put others down, while vulnerable narcissists may act continually victimized, but their motivations are the same. Comparing themselves favorably with other people is how narcissists bolster their inflated sense of self. It's how they prove their superiority, both to themselves and to those around them. These comparisons are often made by the narcissist's critical inner voice.

All people have an "inner critic," or a destructive inner voice that's formed from internalized hurtful experiences. These experiences, and the resulting inner voice, can play a big role in shaping how we view both ourselves and other people. This cruel voice is like an inner coach's dark twin. In most people, the voice of the inner critic is self-destructive, but it can also be self-soothing when its negative appraisals are directed outward.

In narcissists, the voice of the inner critic is almost entirely directed at other people. They don't have a little voice in the back of their mind putting themselves down—instead, that little voice is always putting other people down. They are engaged in a near-constant inner monologue of criticism to make themselves feel better.

For example, if a coworker gets a promotion, they may think something like, "He's such a phony" or "I could do twice the job she does." If they're interested in a romantic partner, the inner critic may say things like, "How could she possibly be interested in anyone else?" or "I'm much better looking than he is." The inner critic also bolsters the narcissist's need to feel special, with thoughts like, "He's wasting his time with her" or "Do something to make them look at you!"

Often, conversations about the narcissist's inner critic are based around whether this inner voice comes from deep wells of insecurity or an inherently inflated sense of self. But I think the more important question to ask is why the narcissist feels the need to listen to these voices in the first place. All of us have the ability to resist our inner critic, so what would be at stake for a narcissist to do the same?

The answer may be found in the narcissist's worldview. Narcissists divide all people into two categories: special and worthless. They hold themselves to this standard as well. They cannot live with the idea that they are no better or worse than anyone else. If they aren't special, then they're nothing. Subsequently, if they don't *feel* special, then they don't feel OK.

The inherent contradiction in the narcissistic worldview is that they believe themselves to be superior, but they are hypersensitive to perceived challenges to that superiority. Their inflated self-image is incredibly fragile because it's just an image—it has no grounding in who they are inside. Such a black-and-white view of the world indicates that, on the inside, the narcissist's sense of self is deeply fragmented. At some point in their lives, they internalized the idea that it's not OK for them to be themselves. As such, they developed a superior external self to protect themselves from the reality of their inherent or authentic self, which they believe to be essentially flawed.

In one case study, a narcissistic patient reported that, when she walked into a room, she automatically went around in her mind, comparing herself to each and every person. When asked to explore the possible roots for such behavior, she recalled her mother comparing her with other girls when she was a child, always telling her that she was the prettiest. This personal reflection conforms to recent studies that indicate narcissism in children is predicted, not by a lack of parental affection, but by parental *over*valuation. Codependency, on the other hand, is the opposite, predicted by a lack of parental warmth. A parent who shows their child special treatment is not necessarily expressing real love or warmth to that child. They may even be compensating for a lack of these feelings in themselves or in the other parent. These parenting techniques do nothing to support a child's authentic sense of self and can actively undermine it, to the point that the child starts to develop narcissistic tendencies (Firestone, 2019).

How People Become Entangled with Narcissists

It's not only codependents that become entangled with narcissists—healthy people often find themselves in increasingly difficult relationships with them, too. As with codependents, the appeal of the narcissist is often a reflection of our own self-esteem. If we are particularly vulnerable to compliments or desire a romantic partner that will make us feel special, that (ironically) makes us more likely to find a narcissist attractive. This need to be "love-bombed" by someone else, in a healthy person, is related to low self-esteem. The apparently confident and cocky narcissist seems like the perfect complement to our insecurity. If we don't have a healthy sense of self-love, then we often have an unhealthy sense of romantic love, too. People who aren't used to giving themselves love find it easier to pour their love into someone else—a dynamic that is perfect for a narcissist. Those with low self-esteem find themselves charmed by the narcissist's grandiose persona and therefore feel privileged and special when the narcissist shows interest in them. The narcissist, of course, feeds off the sense that their partner is starstruck by them and so requires even more devotion and attention.

Of course, narcissists aren't the only ones who put their best foot forward when meeting new people. All of us are predisposed to be a little starstruck when we develop romantic feelings for someone. Feelings of "connection" with someone else can arise from a complex mix of factors. Often, we feel connected with people who make us feel good or bring out the best in us. Though just as often, we feel connected to people who feel familiar, who validate the things we like about ourselves, or who somehow justify qualities that we should objectively be working on. When entering into any romantic partnership, you should always be aware of *why* you feel so good with this person, and if you were to do some serious personal growth, would this person still love the person you're becoming?

Solutions

Knowing all of this, is there anything that a narcissist can do to challenge their inflated sense of self without falling into crisis? Thankfully, the answer is yes.

The first step is for the narcissist to become aware of their inner critic. If they can start to recognize when their inner voices are building them up, they can then start to view this voice as an external commentator rather than an indicator of what they truly think or believe.

But noticing one's inner critic is far from easy. Once the narcissist has spent significant time simply disengaging with their inner critic, they can then start to challenge it with a more realistic view of others and themselves. At this point, they are ready to start exploring where those inner voices may have come from. They can ask themselves questions like:

- Do these voices sound like someone from my past?
- Does the idea of challenging these voices threaten my sense of identity? Why?
- How would I feel if I chose to ignore these voices?

Working with these self-reflective questions can free the narcissist to make changes to their behavior, acting and thinking in ways that are not pre-directed by the inner critic.

A second way for a narcissist to begin coming to terms with their own behavior is to practice self-compassion. Teaching self-compassion to our children is perhaps the most effective way to prevent narcissistic personality disorder. Unlike self-esteem, self-compassion exists outside the narcissism spectrum because it isn't dependent on self-evaluation. Rather, it involves being kind to oneself, treating yourself the same way you would treat a friend or a loved one.

Self-compassion requires taking a mindful approach to one's thoughts and feelings. Mindfulness teaches us not to get overly attached to our thoughts or critical inner voices. Instead, we can acknowledge these attitudes and then let them go. We don't have to let our emotions or destructive thoughts dictate our behaviors if we don't want them to.

But the most important element of self-compassion is the acceptance of the common humanity of all people. To truly accept this, you must let go of the idea that you are somehow different or special. Instead, self-compassion teaches us that every human is worthy in their own way. This worldview is fundamentally opposite the narcissistic worldview and so can be incredibly challenging for a narcissist to come to terms with. Remember that their narcissism exists as a way to compensate for old, deeply painful feelings. Letting go of their self-aggrandizement means having to face these painful feelings. Early in their lives, they were somehow taught that it wasn't OK for them to be themselves. If they do express the desire to challenge their narcissistic traits, self-compassion can be a new, beneficial structure they can use to replace the old, destructive worldview.

Behind the Narcissistic Mask

The narcissistic persona can be extremely charming and charismatic. However, they can just as easily turn entitled and exploitative. Many of us who fall in love with their seductive and exciting energy can be destroyed by their arrogance and aggression. If you don't understand what motivates them, then it can be baffling how someone so engaging can also be so cold and competitive. The better you understand their psychology, the better protected you will be against their inevitable games and lies.

As you now know, narcissists have an inherently impaired sense of self. As such, they think and function very differently from other kinds of people. It's still unclear whether narcissism is more rooted in childhood development or has some kind of genetic component, but what we do know is that narcissistic personality disorder is both deep-rooted and all-pervasive. The severity of the condition, however, varies from person to person. Those with NPD experience these underlying traits with a great level of intensity, but those elsewhere on the spectrum may exhibit more mild versions of the disorder.

Vulnerability

Beneath their strong personalities, narcissists are extremely vulnerable. Psychotherapists consider the narcissistic personality to be extremely emotionally fragile. This is because narcissists suffer from deep-rooted feelings of alienation and emptiness. Beneath their grandiose persona is a toxic level of unconscious shame. Their self-aggrandizement and air of superiority is just a mask that they present to the world—it has nothing to do with who they really are or how they really feel (Lancer, 2019).

The narcissist's craving for power and control can be seen as a direct overcompensation for their extreme vulnerability. They view the expression of vulnerable feelings like fear or shame as a sign of weakness and have no tolerance or respect for people who acknowledge these feelings freely. These defense mechanisms protect them, but they can deeply hurt those around them. As a rule, the more insecure they feel, the more malicious they become.

Shame

Narcissists live with toxic levels of shame. This makes them feel both insecure and inadequate. This is also why they can't tolerate criticism or take responsibility for their actions. Instead, they demand unconditional positive feedback from everyone around them to soothe and quiet this inner shame.

Narcissistic arrogance, then, is just compensation for feelings of inferiority. This arrogance makes them critical and disdainful of other people. They often become bullies, frequently putting down others in order to make themselves feel better.

Shame is also behind narcissistic grandiosity and braggadocio. This is how they convince themselves and others that they excel in everything they do. This is also why they gravitate toward celebrities and other high-status people. Being associated with the best of the best assures them that they're better than other people.

Believe it or not, shame is also behind narcissistic entitlement. Their belief that they deserve to get everything they want is another way to overcompensate for inner feelings of insecurity. Demanding special treatment is how they demonstrate their superiority. If a narcissist's time is more valuable than others', for example, then they shouldn't have to wait in line with everyone else. This is a relatively benign example, but this sense of entitlement can be taken to dangerous extremes. Interpersonal relationships inevitably become parasitic because the narcissist considers their partner to be inherently inferior to them. Worse, they are unable to see themselves as hypocritical or overblown. They genuinely believe that they are superior and therefore special.

Lack of Empathy

Narcissists are extremely limited in their ability to respond to or express an appropriate level of care toward other people's feelings. This is due to their fundamental lack of empathy. They are unable, and often unwilling, to recognize the feelings of others. Recent research has even found that narcissistic brains have characteristic structural abnormalities in the parts of the brain associated with emotions and empathy (Lancer, 2019).

They may say that they love you, but they rarely make you feel loved. Real love requires empathy and compassion—two mental states that are extremely difficult for narcissists to reach. In healthy relationships, each person shows active concern for the other's life and personal growth. We try to understand the experiences of our loved ones, even if they are fundamentally different from our own. Narcissists, on the other hand, are incapable of doing this.

It's this lack of empathy that often leads narcissists to become selfish or hurtful. They view personal relationships as purely transactional. Their primary concern is getting their needs met, not responding to their loved one's feelings. They may feel genuine excitement and passion in the early stages of a romantic partnership, but these feelings are more related to lust than they are to love. Lack of empathy is also what leads narcissists to play emotional games with people. Sacrificing for others is something they are simply not capable of doing. Worse, their lack of empathy desensitizes them to the pain that they may cause those around them.

Emptiness

It's difficult for narcissists to connect with others because they lack a positive emotional connection to themselves. Their underdeveloped sense of self makes them overly dependent on others for validation. Though they project confidence, they secretly fear that they are inherently undesirable. The only way for them to admire themselves is if they see that someone else admires them. This is what drives their craving for constant attention and admiration. Since their sense of self-worth is dependent on what others think, they go to great lengths to control what others think of them. They use personal relationships for self-enhancement rather than true emotional connection. But because they feel so empty on the inside, they are never truly satisfied. No matter what others may do for them, it's never enough. Like emotional vampires, they are constantly seeking to exploit and drain the emotional resources of those around them.

No Boundaries

The term narcissism comes from the story of the Greek hero Narcissus, who infamously fell in love with his own reflection in a pond. At first Narcissus doesn't realize that it's his own reflection he's fallen for—he thinks there's another man looking up at him from the pool. Psychologists gave his name to narcissistic personalities because there's much in the story that seems to correspond with the narcissistic mindset. The significance of someone falling in love with themselves is obvious, but the underlying feelings of emptiness and shame that narcissists experience also distorts their boundaries. Narcissists don't understand other people as separate, fully-formed entities, and instead only see other people as extensions of themselves. Since they have no empathy, they can only conceive of other people as existing to fulfill their needs. It's this view of others that makes them both selfish and totally oblivious to the ways their behavior impacts other people (Lancer, 2019).

Narcissistic Defense Mechanisms

No one likes to feel like a failure. Losing something important, like a test or competition, can strike a hard blow to one's self-esteem. Recent research on failure in the workplace has shown that just the fear of losing can cause leaders to grab for more power and influence than they have necessarily earned (Krauss Whitbourne, 2020).

People experience failure in many different ways. Generally speaking, leaders who are genuinely concerned about the welfare of their group are less devastated by failure than those who are not. People who are primarily concerned with their own personal gain (like narcissists) can feel utterly destroyed by a loss because they can't tolerate feelings of personal inadequacy. It's very difficult to maintain an inflated sense of superiority in the face of failure.

A 2015 study conducted by researchers at the University of Bern sought to examine the way narcissists experience stressful life events. The researchers hypothesized that the narcissist's self-aggrandizing traits could actually cause their own experiences of loss and failure. In other words, because narcissists generally have a negative effect on other people, they would also be more likely to experience negative outcomes throughout their lives. If this were not found to be the case, then the researchers would have to conclude that stressful life events are highly damaging to the narcissist's self-esteem. In this case, losing would theoretically deflate the narcissist's inflated self-image.

A few of the stressful life events monitored by this study were interpersonal problems like rejection by a romantic partner, serious relationship problems, and divorce. The study also monitored experiences like surviving a natural disaster, being the victim of violence, and experiencing the illness of a loved one. After studying more than 600 people, the study ultimately confirmed its hypothesis—narcissists did, indeed, seem to be more likely than other people to experience stressful life events. And despite experiencing these kinds of losses and failures, the narcissists showed no change in the intensity of their narcissism (Krauss Whitbourne, 2020).

What this study shows us is that, while narcissists are more likely to experience failure than other kinds of people, they are less likely to learn from it. Narcissism is considered a "stable" trait, meaning that it does not fluctuate in intensity from day to day. However, no studies have been done to monitor whether or not narcissists experience a brief dip in their narcissistic tendencies immediately after experiencing a failure, before bouncing right back up to their usual levels.

If this were true, the way that a narcissist would regain their grandiosity is by employing one of several defense mechanisms. It's these defenses, including arrogance, contempt, denial, and blaming others for their failures, that make relationships with narcissists so painful and difficult.

Arrogance and contempt. These defenses are employed to inflate the narcissist's ego and shield them from inner feelings of inadequacy. They also relieve the narcissist's feelings of inner shame by projecting them onto the people around them.

Denial. Denial is how narcissists distort their external reality to coincide with their inner fantasies. They distort, rationalize, and twist facts to avoid recognizing anything that might cause them to doubt themselves or question their grandiose persona.

Projection and blame. These strategies allow the narcissist to mentally or verbally assign any of their unpleasant feelings or thoughts to someone else. Blame absolves the narcissist of any personal responsibility for their actions or feelings. In this way, it serves the same purpose as denial. Projection allows the narcissist to believe that any unpleasant feelings or circumstances are solely external and have in no way been caused by something rooted within the narcissist themselves. Unpleasant traits are instead assigned to another person or even another group of people. The narcissist will make you think that you are the one who is selfish and weak when really they are experiencing those traits within themselves. Projection is extremely damaging to the self-esteem of a narcissist's loved ones and can cause serious emotional damage.

Aggression. Pushing others away allows the narcissist to feel safe. Narcissists view the world as hostile and threatening and so perceive all social interactions as a form of conflict. It's this defense that can lead narcissists to become outright abusive, either verbally or physically. Narcissists can be incredibly vindictive and will retaliate against anything they see as disobedience in the people around them.

Envy. Narcissists need to convince themselves that they are the very best. Therefore, it's almost impossible for them to feel happy about someone else's successes. If someone else has something they want, it makes them feel inferior to that person. They have no sense of inherent inner worth, and so their personal value is entirely dependent on external markers of worthiness. Narcissists can be extremely competitive, and their envy can often cause them to act vengefully against those who have what they want. They will not hesitate to sabotage someone else's success and will sometimes act to bring others down out of pure spite. Narcissistic parents, in particular, can become quite envious and even competitive with their children.

Gaslighting. Gaslighting is a form of manipulation designed to make the other person feel like they are imagining things. Gaslighting tactics can be boiled down into three essential phrases (Arabi, 2020):

- That didn't happen.
- You imagined it.
- Are you crazy?

Not everyone's perception of events is identical, and it's actually quite common for two different people to experience the same event very differently. While a healthy person may question, doubt, or contradict your perspective, they will never outright deny it.

Blanket statements. Rather than taking the time to consider things from a new perspective, narcissists tend to generalize other people's opinions. Since they don't consider other people's thoughts to be relevant or interesting, they don't take the time to really listen to what the other person has to say.

Deliberate misrepresentation. When what you're saying doesn't coincide with the narcissist's view of reality, they will intentionally misinterpret what you've said. Rather than taking the time to understand your point of view, they twist your words to give them ridiculous or threatening undertones that weren't originally there.

Threats. Narcissists not only make unreasonable demands on other people's time and energy, but they often seek to punish those who don't live up to their expectations. This threat of punishment can be very subtle, or it can take the form of an outright threat.

Triangulation. This is when someone invokes the opinions or perspectives of another person in order to validate their own feelings in a social interaction. This tactic is used by abusive people of all kinds to both validate the abuser's behavior and invalidate the victim's response to said behavior.

Being the know-it-all. Narcissists seek to position themselves as the expert on any given topic by repeatedly invalidating other people's opinions or perspectives. They don't simply disagree with others— they seek to demonstrate that the other person doesn't know what they're talking about (Ni, 2019).

Understanding where these defense mechanisms come from can help you to protect yourself against them. These defenses can appear in more mild forms in those with narcissistic tendencies, but they can reach dangerous and abusive levels in people with NPD. Learning to spot these problematic behaviors will both give you a level of clarity and help you to make sure your needs are also being met in the relationship. As the parent guardian of a potential narcissist, the question you're probably most eager to answer is this: How do people become narcissists in the first place?

Chapter 3:

Narcissism in Children

Technically, it's impossible for a child to be diagnosed with narcissistic personality disorder. However, narcissistic tendencies can and do start to appear in early childhood. The biggest difficulty in spotting these tendencies is the simple fact that small children are selfish. This is a very normal part of early development. All young children are primarily concerned with getting their own needs; their brains simply aren't sophisticated enough to understand that other people have needs, too. Children maintain this self-centeredness into their teens, which aids them as they struggle to find independent identities from their parents.

In a healthy person, childhood self-centeredness eventually falls away as the brain develops, and the teenager starts to have formative interpersonal experiences. Empathy is something that should develop in childhood, and its absence is a strong predictor for developing a personality disorder as an adult.

However, because even healthy teenagers are typically self-centered and aren't quite socially sophisticated enough to be good manipulators, psychologists are very hesitant to diagnose NPD in people below the age of

18. As a parent, it's your job to watch for early warning signs of the disorder in your child, with the intention of intervening before it can develop into adulthood. Children can show red flags and narcissistic predictors as young as age two. However, this is extremely early in a child's development. With the right intervention, parents can guide the child to learn how to become accountable for their own actions or how to have empathy for others.

The older a person gets, the more resistant they are to treatment for their narcissism. Narcissism can be a particularly difficult disorder to correct because it's in the nature of the disorder for a person to be unable to think critically about themselves. In order to spot the warning signs of narcissism in young children, we first have to understand what healthy childhood development should look like.

Selfishness is often the marker that people look for, but this can be misleading. All children and teenagers are inherently selfish or at least more selfish than healthy adults. But the only way for children to let go of this selfishness is to develop healthy and lasting levels of self-esteem. Children with healthy self-esteems believe that they are loved and worthy of love. Self-esteem and self-centeredness are very different, in the sense that cultivating a high self-esteem doesn't justify prioritizing one's needs to the detriment of others (Johnson, 2017).

Over the course of a child's development, their self-centeredness will slowly give way to self-esteem. To become adults who are mentally well, children must learn how to consider other people's perspectives and develop empathy for other people's suffering. Healthy children begin to demonstrate that they genuinely care about other people's feelings. Not developing this empathy is one of the biggest warning signs, not only of narcissism, but for any personality disorder.

We now know how adults with NPD can be expected to act. At this point, you are familiar with the condition's diagnostic criteria. Their lack of empathy is demonstrated both in their words and their actions. They maintain grandiose beliefs of superiority and believe that they are special. They are arrogant, self-important, haughty, and obsessed with fantasies of unlimited success or power. They are entitled and require excessive admiration. They exploit or take advantage of people for personal gain. They pit people against each other to get what they want. They are envious of others and seek to sabotage others by preying on negative emotions. We also know that they have a long list of defense mechanisms and manipulative techniques at their disposal.

Those who find themselves in close relationships with narcissists often question their sanity and experience high levels of anxiety. In short, narcissistic adults tend to make other people feel utterly miserable. They can become extremely aggressive with people who don't agree with or outright admire them. This is hardly the kind of person any parent wants their child to grow into. To make things even more difficult, adults diagnosed with NPD are extremely resistant to treatment, as they are unable to understand that something might be wrong with them (Johnson, 2017).

But these behaviors are all associated with narcissistic *adults*. Narcissistic traits in children tend to manifest themselves in slightly different ways. Instead, warning signs of narcissism in teenagers and children tend to look something like this (Narcissist Abuse Support, 2019):

Entitlement

Many children get the message early in life that they are entitled to have whatever they want. The small child may demand a new toy, regardless of its cost. A teenager may show entitlement in their actions, believing they are allowed to see their friends whenever they want or say what they want to anyone without regard for that person's feelings. Young adults may demand that their parents pay their bills or bail them out if they get into trouble. As they mature into adulthood, they will start actively seeking out people who are willing to tolerate this kind of behavior, giving into their demands and giving them whatever they ask for.

Inflated Ego

Though many parents worry that craving for attention on social media is a sign of self-absorption, true egotistical behavior is much more sinister than a desire to keep up with the other kids. If other kids are mean or otherwise challenge their social image, all children will experience some level of hurt. A narcissistic ego will take this one step further—the child will seek revenge on the children that caused their wound. Budding covert narcissists are even more subtle. They may not demand attention from people on social media, but they demand unconditional loyalty from everyone around them. In fact, demands for attention in real life are much more indicative of developing narcissism than demands for attention online.

In fact, most parents who express concern about narcissistic behaviors in their child often cite things like taking selfies or spending excessive amounts of time on social media. But these are not indicators of narcissism, and indeed, may not be indicators of any problematic development in your child. For contemporary children, social media is a primary way in which they connect with their peers, just as talking on the phone was for children of the previous generation. Needing to take the perfect selfie may be causing problems for your child, but narcissism probably isn't one of them. Narcissistic online behavior manifests when your child begins to intentionally hurt others for their own personal gain or status.

Lack of Empathy

Just as in adults, a noticeable lack of empathy is a big indicator of narcissism in children. Pay attention to the ways in which your child seeks attention from you or other members of the family. A narcissistic child will display no regard for anyone's feelings but their own. They won't want to hear about your day or be able to sit still through a sibling's hockey game. Your life and the lives of other members of the family hold no importance or value to them. They may find ways to lead every conversation back to themselves.

Pathological Lying

Even healthy teenagers tend to lie a lot, but narcissistic children tell lies without regard for the harm they may cause others. A narcissistic teenager seeking revenge or negative attention might tell people at school that her father molested her or that his mother is emotionally abusive. In fact, lies about physical abuse or alcoholism in the home are actually quite common in narcissistic teens. Most teenagers lie about where they were at night, but narcissists will tell long, detailed stories that are both sophisticated and difficult to refute. Don't be fooled by details. A clear answer to your question doesn't necessarily make it true. Make sure to follow up on your teenager's story if you suspect them of trying to gaslight you.

Desperate for Attention

All children like to be the center of attention. Narcissists will do anything to both win your approval and make themselves look better than their siblings. In school, they will either play the know-it-all, constantly needing to prove to the teacher how smart they are, or play the class clown, creating chaos and constantly breaking the rules. For the narcissistic child, attention is attention, so they will do whatever it takes to get it.

Manipulation

All children will pull on your heartstrings if they think it will get them what they want. Narcissistic children will take this a step further and attempt to make you feel guilty if you don't respond to their charms. They learn very quickly what tactics work and will often play parents or guardians against one another in order to get what they want.

Tantrums

Again, all little children have tantrums, but narcissistic children have much less control over their emotions than is developmentally appropriate. If your child has regular tantrums beyond the age of three, this is a warning sign for developing narcissism.

Uncooperative

Narcissistic children don't get along well with others. They feel that they are somehow better than their peers. Their relationships with other children are based primarily on what the other child can do for them. Any friendships are superficial, and friends that they can't control are discarded. Pay close attention to the quality of your child's relationships, because on the surface, narcissistic children tend to look like they have a big circle of friends. But are these intimate connections, or is your child slowly building a circle of admirers? A big warning sign is if your child wishes to make friends with someone because it will increase their social status.

The Princess and the Bully

Narcissistic children tend to go one of two ways at school—they strive to be the most attractive, popular, and smartest student in the school or they become vicious and feared bullies. Aggression and persistent boundary breaking are also red flags for developing narcissism.

Victim Mentality

Children with narcissistic traits have a tendency to view themselves as perpetual victims. All negative outcomes seem to happen "to" them. Any kind of bad behavior, like stealing or cheating, is justified by external pressures or other people "making" them do it.

Aggressive Behaviors

Dangerously difficult or demanding behaviors are most certainly a red flag and should be taken seriously.

Laying Blame

Narcissistic children always find someone else to blame for their own bad behaviors. They are never wrong and never admit to being wrong, even when directly confronted by an adult. They can sometimes concoct very elaborate (and convincing) stories in order to shift the blame onto someone else if they get in trouble.

Creating Drama

Narcissistic children will intentionally incite chaos or conflict simply for the excitement of it. While healthy children dislike conflict in the home, narcissistic children thrive on it.

Never Following Rules

All children take a special delight in doing things they aren't supposed to do. Narcissistic children take it one step further, behaving as if the rules simply don't apply to them.

Stealing

A major indicator of narcissism in a child is frequent stealing, especially at a young age. This thieving stems from the belief that they are entitled to have whatever they want, even if it belongs to someone else. As adults, this behavior often shows up again in marriages or roommate situations—what belongs to them is theirs, and what belongs to everyone else in the household is also theirs.

Inability to Accept Failure

Failure is just as hard for children as it is for adults. But narcissistic children simply cannot accept the fact that failure is a necessary part of the learning process. A child that will do anything to win, including cheating or stealing, is displaying early signs of narcissistic behavior.

There is much debate about how much of NPD is biological and how much is due to problems in childhood development. However, what we do know for sure is that the circumstances of childhood do have some degree of influence on whether or not a child grows up to be a narcissist. Empathy is something that young children have to be taught. In many cases, parents do their best to teach their children core values, and those children still behave badly. When this happens, loving parents tend to put a lot of blame and shame on themselves, but this often leads to problematic parenting styles like neglecting, indulgence, and coldness, all of which have been linked with narcissism.

Instead, if you notice your child showing two or more of these qualities, ask yourself the question: Can they change? Remember that every child is different, and the dynamics within every family are different. The age at which a child starts to exhibit these traits is also an important factor in a parent's ability to effectively intervene. Once a narcissistic child reaches adulthood, there's often very little anyone can do to help them change their ways. Because there are so many interconnecting factors, there is no one right way to "fix" narcissistic behaviors in children. Instead, the approach taken by you, your co-parent, and other adults in your child's life should be tailored to your child's specific needs. That being said, there are some general ways that you can intervene, including (Johnson, 2017):

- Teach your child empathy.
- Teach them to value character traits like honesty and kindness.
- Actively challenge entitled attitudes.
- Actively challenge greed.
- Routinely ask them to put other people before themselves.
- Work to bolster their self-esteem.
- Don't allow them to blame other people for their own problems.

In addition to positive interventions, you can also actively teach your teenagers about narcissism and how to recognize it in other people. This intervention will be less effective in young children, however, as it requires the ability to think critically about other people's behaviors.

Teaching teenagers about narcissism can not only help them to watch for its toxic signs within themselves but protect them from narcissistic people in the future. Short of this, simply teaching your children the difference between lies and truths can save them from succumbing to manipulative people in the future.

Above all, the best protection against narcissism is instilling your child with healthy self-esteem. If you're not sure how to accomplish this (or why what you're currently doing doesn't seem to be working) don't hesitate to reach out to parenting resources or professionals for guidance.

Healthy Childhood Behavior vs. Narcissistic Behavior

If you suspect narcissistic tendencies in your child, it's very important to remember that egocentric traits are a very healthy and normal part of early childhood development. This quality even plays an important role in adolescence, helping teenagers to form their own identities, separate from their parents. Think about the teenager who screams, "You never do anything for me!" after you've just spent a few hundred dollars on her field hockey equipment. Or who refuses to clean the bathroom because it's "not his job." Both of these are examples of teenage narcissism. As maddening as these situations can be, they are examples of *normal* teenage narcissism. These kinds of incidents are not necessarily a reflection of your parenting style or the quality of your child's life. All teenagers go through a phase of believing that the world does (or should) revolve around them. But as your child gets older, you should start to see their capacity for empathy slowly expand.

Narcissism, then, can be particularly difficult to spot in children for the simple reason that all children are narcissistic. In healthy children, that narcissism is a necessary part of their development, one that helps them to learn and grow at a normal rate. In narcissistic children, however, their narcissistic traits begin to impair the quality of their relationships and even start to cause problems in school.

A little less than 6% of all adults have narcissistic personality disorder. All people under the age of 18 display at least normal levels of childhood narcissism, which is why therapists very rarely make this diagnosis in children. The same behaviors that would be considered "narcissistic" in an adult are quite normal and even healthy in a child.

The question, of course, is how to find the line between healthy teenage egocentrism and pre-narcissistic personality traits. There are also different expressions of narcissism that are appropriate in young children but are problematic if they last into adolescence (Morin, 2020).

There are a few characteristics of normal childhood narcissism that, while occasionally frustrating, do not necessarily indicate any problems in your childhood development. These characteristics include (Jana, 2014):

Overconfident Self-Beliefs

It's very normal for preschoolers to have an inflated and fantastical understanding of their own abilities, an understanding that is likely to have no grounding in reality. This overestimation is actually an important part of childhood, as it gives young children the confidence they need to take risks and explore the world without feeling crippled by the limits of their real abilities. Beyond the preschool age, however, healthy children need to start developing a more realistic awareness of their accomplishments and abilities. This is best achieved by recognizing the connection between effort and outcome.

Craving Attention

Young children have naturally grandiose expectations of attention and affection of their parents, but adequate fulfillment of these needs is critical to the development of a child's self-esteem. As they grow, it's important to instill your child with healthy self-talk that will bring them resilience in the face of failure.

Entitlement

Young children often exhibit their personal autonomy through entitled behaviors. Taking (or sometimes demanding) what they want is the only way for young children to exert any kind of control over what happens to them.

Limited Empathy

Humans aren't inherently wired for empathy. The wider range of emotions your child is allowed to feel as a child, the easier it will be to recognize and understand those emotions in other people.

To summarize, a healthy child will:

- crave attention, but express gratitude and appreciation for the attention they receive.
- aspire to unrealistic heights of achievement or role-play as magical beings, but can tell the difference between pretend play and real life.
- demand that their needs be met, but those needs are both realistic and fulfillable by their parents.
- show an early ability to both make friends and get along with other members of the family.

By contrast, a narcissistic child will (Cunha, 2020):

- assume that any attention they receive is somehow owed them, and never seem to be satisfied, no matter how much attention they get.
- believe that they are superior and that other children are somehow beneath them.
- have unreasonable expectations and develop needs that are impossible for their parents to satisfy.
- find it difficult to either make or maintain close friendships.

If your child displays two or more of the following traits, your child may be at risk for developing NPD later in life (Specialist, 2020):

- exhibits extreme feelings of self-importance.
- has a fantastical self-image that includes unlimited achievements and power.
- feels entitled to have anything they want.
- experiences gaze aversion, or is uncomfortable with eye contact.
- suffers with extreme separation anxiety.
- engages in play that is pathologic or outright harmful.
- believes that they are somehow better than other children.
- demands extremely high levels of respect and adoration.
- is an extreme opportunist.
- shows inability to recognize that other people have needs.
- is arrogant.
- has a tendency to exaggerate their personal abilities or achievements.
- is extremely exploitative.
- is extremely envious of other people's things or achievements.
- seems strangely formal, even in personal or close relationship settings.
- is unable to take constructive criticism.
- blames others for their failures, bad behaviors, or negative emotions.

A child that displays one or two of these traits may still be developing normally. The more of these traits your child exhibits, the more at risk they are for NPD. Consider this case study. Dave is 11-years-old. He and a school friend are comparing toy cars that they got for Christmas. Dave's friend's car is visibly more expensive than his own. In a rage, he breaks his friend's car. When his mom reprimands him later, he insists that he did nothing wrong and refuses to accept any kind of discipline. He even blames his friend for the incident, insisting that his friend should not have shown him the car in the first place.

In this story, we see several warning signs for NPD. Jealousy and envy are emotions that all humans experience, and ones that children experience quite intensely. The kind of envy that Dave exhibits in the story, however, goes far beyond wishing that his toy was as good as his friend's. Dave flies into a rage at the very idea that his friend might own something better than he does, which hardly fits the criteria for supportive friendship. While healthy children typically understand why they're in trouble when they get caught doing something wrong, Dave seems to genuinely not understand why he's in trouble. Instead, he insists that it was his friend's fault and that his friend should have known better. This kind of deflection is called "victim blaming," and it displays a serious lack of boundaries. By insisting that his friend should have "known better," Dave is insisting that his friend is responsible for taking care of his feelings. He, on the other hand, has no clear regard for the feelings of his friend.

But how do children develop narcissistic tendencies in the first place? The answer, unfortunately, is still unknown. However, psychologists have been able to link certain early childhood experiences, environmental conditions, and underlying physiological conditions to the development of narcissism and NPD in adults. These predictors can be divided into three basic categories, as developed by James F. Masterson: nature, nurture, and fate.

Nature, according to Masterson, is a person's innate temperament. It's the set of personality traits that we are born with and that are either strengthened or suppressed throughout our lives. Studies have found that children who are naturally more dramatic, aggressive, or attention-seeking were much more likely to develop NPD than children with different personality traits, even when raised in similar conditions (Greenberg, 2020).

Nurture is where parenting comes in. This is how parents and other adults treat a child early in life, shaping their behaviors and attitudes as they grow into adulthood. There are a few different parenting styles and household dynamics that have been linked by psychologists to the development of NPD in adults (Gross, 2015):

Negligent Parenting

Though more closely related to codependency than to narcissism, many adults who are diagnosed with NPD report having parents who were cold, detached, or somehow unresponsive to their care when they were children.

Codependent Parenting

Codependent parents frequently cross the line between protective and overprotective, love and obsession, and therefore fail to teach their children healthy boundaries or instill in them a healthy self-esteem.

Excessive Pampering

Overvaluation of children can directly contribute to the formation of narcissistic tendencies. Rather than increasing their self-esteem, teaching your child that they are entitled to special treatment causes them to develop a narcissistic view of themselves. Many narcissists report having parents who were overvaluing or who treated them as the "golden child" of the family. Common remembrances are of parents who were overprotective or extremely lenient when it came to childhood discipline (Van Schie, Jarman, Huxley, & Grenyer, 2020).

Narcissistic Parenting

Children raised with a narcissistic value system are, unsurprisingly, more likely to grow up to be narcissists themselves. All children wish to please their parents and wish to avoid being rebuked or punished. Most see their parents as god-like, all-knowing figures, at least until they hit puberty. This provides the perfect source of unending, unconditional attention for a narcissistic parent.

Many children of narcissistic parents develop covert or vulnerable narcissism, as their parents often punish them when they try to take the spotlight or assert their individuality. Many others become communal narcissists, learning to feel special by pleasing others.

Almost every child who grows up in a narcissistic household, whether they become narcissists or not, tend to develop an extremely critical inner voice. As such, children of narcissists are just as likely to become codependent as they are to have full-blown NPD (Greenberg, 2017).

Excessive Criticism

Constant or harsh criticism from parents can make children feel inadequate and crush their self-esteem and subsequently develop narcissism as a defense mechanism against these feelings.

Adoption or Divorced Parents

Children who are adopted or whose parents get divorced before the age of 5 rarely experience these events as a trauma. But children whose parents die or divorce between the ages of 5 and 8 often fail to get the love that they need from their parents or guardians and so develop excessive self-love to compensate.

Irrational Expectations

We all want our children to succeed. Placing incredibly high expectations on your children can either make them feel too highly or too poorly about themselves, both of which can lead to the development of narcissism.

Abuse

Whether emotional or physical, childhood abuse makes people feel victimized and unloved. As a defense, the child may develop feelings of superiority and inflated self-love. Many people with NPD grew up in abusive households.

Narcissistic Extension

When parents see their children as extensions of themselves, they start to idealize the child, pinning their own sense of self-worth and accomplishment on the child. These kinds of children almost inevitably grow up to feel special or believe that they have special talents that other children don't have.

Alcoholism

The children of alcoholic parents are also at high risk for developing NPD later in life. The children of addicts often find themselves struggling for attention from their parents or other members of the family. As with children of abusive parents, these children often learn that the only way to keep the peace is to please their parents. This, in turn, teaches them that love is something that must be earned.

Shame-Based Parenting

Children who are frequently shamed by their parents, especially about their inner worlds, are at risk for NPD. Shame in children can either make them withdraw emotionally from others or make them grandiose in order to overcompensate for their perceived weaknesses. Either reaction sets them up to develop narcissistic personality traits when they get older (Walansky, 2020).

Hypersensitivity

If they are not taught how to manage their feelings, hypersensitive children can sometimes develop narcissism as a way to avoid having to think about the outside world.

Genetics

While it's still unclear whether or not NPD is a genetic condition, it does seem to be connected to certain genetic sequences and physiological abnormalities in the brain.

Culture

Believe it or not, studies have also shown that certain cultures and societies are more likely to produce narcissists than others. In general, collectivist societies, ones that value the group over the individual, see much lower rates of NPD than individualist societies. For example, children raised in New York, a notoriously competitive place, are four times more likely to develop NPD as adults than children raised in Iowa (Webber, 2016).

Finally, **fate** describes chance events that happen in early childhood and that have a formative impact on the way that children will grow up to view themself and the world. The first three years of a child's life are particularly important for development. It's during this stage of life that children learn to separate and individuate themselves from their mother. If their mother is absent during this stage, whether physically or emotionally, it can have profoundly negative consequences for the child's development unless another maternal figure like a grandmother or an aunt steps in to fill a similar role (Greenberg, 2020).

If you do suspect your child may have narcissistic traits, the first thing to do is reach out to a childhood psychologist who specializes in personality disorders. The therapist will first make an initial evaluation of the child's mental health. They will talk with your child, determining your child's levels of self-love and sense of importance. The therapist will also evaluate the child's behavior toward them, making note of whether the child is condescending, polite, anxious, or forthcoming. If necessary, the therapist may recommend a physical examination, or even a brain scan, to rule out any potential physical or neurological causes for the child's behaviors.

After the initial evaluation, the therapist will draft a mental health care plan that is specifically tailored to your child's needs and behaviors. The therapist may ask your child to complete questionnaires, assessments, or scale tests to help them make a more accurate diagnosis. They may ask your child questions about their personal life, such as their academic performance, the quality of their friendships, or how many friends they have. Remember that there are many other conditions that can look similar to narcissistic personality disorder in children, such as hypomania, codependency, and psychopathy. The therapist will want to rule out any of these other conditions, paying close attention to whether your child's narcissistic traits are consistent or mood-based (Jana, 2014).

Much literature on narcissism and other personality disorders will tell you that these conditions cannot be cured. While this is technically true, they can certainly be managed, especially with early intervention. The most effective treatment for NPD is some form of psychotherapy. There are no medications for treating narcissism, but since many narcissists suffer from depression or anxiety, the doctor may prescribe your child with an antidepressant (Jana, 2014).

It's critically important for you and your child to follow the treatment steps recommended by the doctor to avoid problems in the future. Many teenagers and young adults with untreated narcissism can develop comorbid problems that are much more difficult to treat, such as:

- addictive disorders.
- relationship crises.
- social awkwardness.
- difficult relationships at school or at home.

In addition to the treatment plan prescribed by your therapist, there are a few things you can do to help manage your child's narcissism at home. Narcissistic children need to be explicitly taught healthy emotional and relationship dynamics, which can be done in the following ways (Hammond, 2019):

Be Firm, Never Violent

Violence and aggression at home will only serve to further emotionally alienate your child from you. Narcissists have an inflated ego and so will take any discipline personally. Remember that they have extremely fragile self-esteem. Continue to discipline your child when necessary, but use methods that are practical and mindful of your child's self-esteem.

Curb Entitled Behaviors

Make it clear to your child that they will not get special treatment over other members of the family. If your child behaves in a bossy way with their siblings or friends, teach them that it's not OK to bully others. Make sure not to ridicule or excessively criticize.

Moderate Your Conversations

Teach your child how to listen. Tell them that during any conversation, they should listen half the time and speak half the time. Practise at home with them.

Balance Relationships

Teach your child that they must be considerate toward others in the family in order for there to be a healthy family dynamic. Demonstrate to them how you and your co-parent share responsibilities, working together to care for the family.

Love Unconditionally

Do not give or withhold love based on your child's achievements. Don't reward them with gifts and privileges when they succeed or insult and ridicule them when they fail. Instead, praise them for their successes, and comfort them after failures, demonstrating to them that your love for them is unconditional.

Narcissism is not a disease and doesn't have to be a problem. Remember, all of us need a certain amount of narcissism to be considered healthy. It's only when our narcissistic traits begin to damage our relationships or quality of life that it starts to become a problem. Though managing your child's narcissism can be difficult and time-consuming, it is absolutely worth it in the end.

Is it Narcissism?

Narcissism is far from the only psychological disorder that can appear in childhood. In 2008, researchers at Boston University estimated that as much as 10% of children in the United States have the common cold at any given time. And much more recently, the CDC found that the same percentage of children in the United States (about 10%) are diagnosed with attention deficit hyperactivity disorder (ADHD).

In fact, ADHD appears to be on the rise. Compare these numbers to 1970, when just 1% of American children had an ADHD diagnosis. This number rose to 5% by 1980, though this rise could arguably be attributed to an increase in education and ADHD awareness. But by 1995, those numbers had shot up as high as 17% in some school districts.

These kinds of numbers are cause for concern. Some of the major symptoms· of childhood ADHD include difficulty listening, forgetfulness, and distractibility. Some psychologists have argued that, to a certain degree, these are challenges that all children have. Unwillingness to finish difficult tasks or excessive talking could be signs of ADHD, but they could also be signs that a child is simply not emotionally mature.

For these and other reasons, there has been a recent evaluation by the psychological community into the ways we diagnose ADHD in children. For the most part, children with ADHD do not get a sensitive or sophisticated evaluation before being diagnosed. Most parents reach out to pediatricians about their child's behaviors, not to therapists or psychologists. While many pediatricians are qualified to give an ADHD diagnosis, the average visit with a pediatrician is less than thirty minutes—hardly enough time to make a thorough evaluation (Gnaulati, 2013).

It's also true, however, that contemporary parents are much more aware of ADHD and its warning signs than parents of the past. While this education is valuable, it can sometimes lead parents to miss other warning signs in their children's behavior or misread certain behaviors. If your child is distractible or hyperactive, they could very well have ADHD. But that's not the *only* thing those behaviors indicate.

Unfortunately, this combination of parental awareness and brief clinical visits may very well result in premature ADHD diagnoses. For parents who are unfamiliar with a psychological evaluation, the brevity and speed with which their child is diagnosed may even be a relief. Knowing what the problem is may make them feel more empowered to help their child.

But what does all this have to do with narcissism?

For starters, what many parents don't realize is that there are a number of overlaps between ADHD and NPD warning signs. Overconfident self-appraisals and craving recognition from others are narcissistic traits, but they can fuel ADHD-like behaviors, such as an inability to wait for one's turn or even to sit still. Even normal levels of childhood narcissism can be mistaken for ADHD by parents who just don't know what they're looking at. ADHD children often have meltdowns if they can't solve a difficult problem—but so do narcissistic children. High emotionality is a feature of ADHD, but it can also be a narcissistic indicator. Problematic behaviors don't necessarily indicate either condition. Stirring up drama is just as much a feature of normal childhood narcissism as it is a warning sign of future NPD. So is craving attention or lying to get out of trouble.

ADHD children have problems with executive functioning, which makes it difficult for them to complete assignments on time or remember deadlines. But the inability to complete assignments can also come from narcissism. Your child may believe that the deadlines simply don't apply to them or that they're too smart for homework. Alternatively, your child may have other reasons for not completing their work on time, such as a chaotic household or low self-esteem.

Many children are picky eaters. This is most likely due to the fact that children have more taste buds than adults. ADHD children can sometimes throw tantrums or refuse to eat certain foods because they feel overstimulated. Narcissistic children can refuse to eat what's in front of them because they feel entitled to eat whatever they want. Again, the same behavior can have multiple underlying causes.

ADHD children also need a great deal of structure in their lives. They struggle to do well with open activities or function normally in chaotic environments. Narcissistic children can also act out in open-ended activities in order to make themselves the center of attention. Healthy children can sometimes throw tantrums or misbehave as a way to signal to the adults in the room that they feel overwhelmed.

Far more parents reach out to professionals because they suspect their child has ADHD, not narcissism. Since the core symptoms of ADHD so closely resemble normal, healthy childhood narcissism, many children may find themselves misdiagnosed. Since ADHD is a more common disorder, its diagnosis is handed out much more frequently and isn't examined as closely as rarer conditions like narcissism, bipolar, or autism.

To make things more complicated, many narcissistic traits in young children are a perfectly normal part of their development. Young children, as we know, tend to drastically overestimate their abilities or even convince themselves that they have magical powers. It's very normal for preschool children to have an optimistic and overconfident view of their physical and mental abilities. It's only the intervention of stubborn or restrictive parents that prevents young children from actually believing that they can drive cars or use power tools by themselves. Young children have not yet developed the ability to distinguish between knowing about something and actually experiencing it.

We expect preschool children to have big, even fantastical ideas about their own abilities. A recent survey conducted by the University of California, Los

Angeles, found that most first graders will answer "yes" to the question, "Are you one of the smartest kids in your class?" If you've ever watched young children play, you'll see them taking on super-personas or giving themselves superpowers. This overconfidence in young children gives them the courage that they need to explore a world that is still relatively new to them (Gnaulati, 2013).

As children progress through elementary school, however, these fantastical self-beliefs will start to align more closely with their actual abilities. They will start to learn the relationship between work, commitment, and positive outcomes. The way that parents respond to their children's demonstrations of their supposed talents, whether successful or not, will have a significant impact on a child's ability to accurately assess their own abilities.

For example, imagine that your child has a meltdown if they can't easily finish a difficult task. He gives the problem the smallest amount of effort before falling to pieces. This could be a symptom of ADHD. Children with ADHD can have difficulty retaining the information required to complete a problem or complex assignment. But if this child is in elementary school, it's equally likely that they still possess the narcissistic trait of optimistic self-appraisals. He still believes that his power is unlimited and that simply knowing about a task is enough to achieve it. Your child's tantrums in the face of hard work may also be an indicator of low self-esteem. He may be extremely productive when working through tasks he knows he can complete, motivated by the praise he knows he will receive from parents and teachers. This makes him feel accomplished and good about himself. But it doesn't teach him the relationship between hard work and positive outcomes. So when he's faced with work that is challenging, he shuts down. He feels like a failure because he still believes that he should automatically be good at everything he does. He doesn't understand that having to work at something doesn't reflect badly on one's intelligence or abilities.

Though often cited as evidence for ADHD, wild swings in productivity are more often than not related to shaky self-esteem. These children pin their sense of self-worth on praise and admiration from others and haven't yet learned how to work hard in the face of failure. When they succeed, their self-esteem soars, and when they fail, they fall into a terrible depression.

Parental responses to childhood successes and failures also have a big impact on how much attention the child needs. Bragging and showing off in young children is one of the major ways in which they acquire self-esteem. This idea was brought into public awareness in the 1980s when Dr. Heinz Kohut published a series of formative papers about narcissism. He was one of the first to insist that the way a parent handles a child's exhibitionistic tendencies in early childhood was central to the formation of that child's sense of self-worth (Gnaulati, 2013). For example, think about a baby taking her first, unassisted steps. Her smile is big. Her mood is bright. She looks up at her parents, and specifically at their faces, expecting to see her pride and happiness mirrored back at her. The appreciation and joy she receives from her parents during this and other exhibitionistic moments will form an important part of the child's self-experience. The praise she does (or doesn't) receive from her parents during this critical time will form her sense of self-worth in the future.

Of course, not all childhood exhibitionistic displays end in success. Your child may swing flawlessly across the monkey bars, only to collapse when he tries to execute a cartwheel across the grass. Even the most loving parents can't always provide the undivided or sensitive attention that their child needs in the moment. But most importantly, parents should not be a constant source of praise in a young child's life. Instead, parents should make an effort to recognize and appreciate their child's talents or successes. When that child inevitably fails, it's important not to perform any emotional rescuing. Gushing or fawning when a child's pride is wounded should be avoided.

For example, imagine your 7-year-old loses a footrace with a neighbor. It can be tempting to say something encouraging, like "Don't worry, honey. You're a great runner! Dad even thinks you could be in the Olympics one day!" Don't. Instead, try something like, "I'm sorry that you lost the race, honey. You must be feeling pretty bad right now. Losing never feels good. Did you know that [the other child] has been playing soccer all summer? He's been practicing his running for months! It would be tough for anyone to race him right now. If you want to make your legs stronger, why don't you start jogging with Dad on Sunday mornings?" This kind of response helps your child to take a more realistic view of his abilities. But it does so while instilling in him the kind of healthy self-talk he needs to build resilience in the face of future failures.

Parents tend to find overconfidence in their children tolerable and sometimes even cute. As such, expression of entitlement is typically the narcissistic warning sign that most parents see first. This, too, is a normal part of childhood development. Consider the child who refuses to eat the dinner you've prepared for him and the family or the child who runs off down the driveway when you try to get her into the car for her doctor's appointment. These displays may be maddening, but they are hardly abnormal. Temper tantrums are one of the only ways young children have to control what happens to or around them. They are also a way for your child to communicate with you that they've been under or overstimulated and need a change. This is why young children tend to display difficult behaviors when there's a lot of activity in the house. Think about the rush to get your children packed off to school in the morning. Defiant behaviors at this point in the day may simply be your child's way of signaling to you that they feel overwhelmed by all the activity.

Lack of empathy is arguably the most problematic feature of narcissism in adults. But young children are still developing this profoundly emotional quality. Empathy is the ability to recognize and understand the feelings of other people. It helps us to become more connected with others and sensitive to their needs. A preschooler may hover awkwardly near a crying friend, unsure how to comfort them. The fact that they display some kind of emotional connection or sensitivity to their friend's feelings is key. As they get older, their caring behaviors will become more natural and sophisticated. By about age five, most children can name the feelings that the people around them are experiencing. The more emotions a child is allowed to experience themselves, the better they will be at recognizing those feelings in someone else.

Healthy levels of empathy are perhaps one of the most important indicators of a child's psychological well-being. Children have to learn how to recognize intense feelings like distress or anger in other people without becoming overwhelmed or desensitized to them. Just as children can develop a lack of empathy, they can also develop too much of it, becoming completely overwhelmed when other people display intense emotions. Ironically, this kind of response can also be a predictor of narcissism, as the over sensitized child will start to focus more on protecting themselves from other people's emotions than they do on comforting or caring for others (Gnaulati, 2013).

Someone who has a great deal of empathy for others is "ruthful." Someone who has a noticeable lack of empathy we call "ruthless." Ruthful people are able to experience someone else's suffering as their own. This prevents them from becoming overly aggressive in conflicts, as the pain they inflict on others hurts them, too. This sensitivity is what prevents people from committing overly violent or aggressive acts against others. It's empathy that motivates us to back off during heated arguments and make up with loved ones after conflict. Empathy isn't necessarily something that humans are wired for. Some children pick it up more easily, but others need to be prompted to think about the feelings of others. "How do you think he/she/they feel?" is a great question to ask your young child, especially if their bad behaviors have inflicted emotional pain on someone else. Empathy is also what helps us to sacrifice our own needs for the needs of others. Gently remind your child that, on Suzie's birthday, it's time to pay attention to Suzie, or ask them to bring some food into Grandma's room when she's not feeling well.

Teaching yourself about the normal expressions of narcissism in children will not only help you to spot the warning signs of clinical narcissism, but it can also help you to more accurately determine if your child's behaviors are due to another underlying disorder.

Chapter 4:

Dealing with the

Narcissistic Child

Family dynamics can unintentionally protect or even encourage narcissistic children. Parents often accidentally misplace their anger about narcissistic behaviors onto something or someone else. Families can even become fearful of the narcissist's rage or disapproval, often going to great lengths to keep the narcissist satisfied. An abusive outburst is often minimized by the family, pretending that it simply didn't happen or insisting to other family members that it wasn't that bad.

People with narcissistic family members often don't understand just how dysfunctional their family dynamics have become until they have something to compare their experience with. Parents don't always know what behaviors are healthy and which are cause for concern. And even when they do, they may not know the right way to handle such behaviors.

When families don't know what they're dealing with, they often inadvertently begin to protect the narcissist.

Behaviors that are harmful and hurtful start to be excused. The narcissist's rationalizing of their behavior becomes more and more acceptable to other members of the family. The more the narcissist gets away with, the more adept they become at manipulating and shifting blame.

Recognizing dysfunction can be very difficult when you are embroiled in it. These are some common dynamics to watch for in your own family, as these are all ways that people can inadvertently start protecting the narcissist in their life (Hammond, 2019b):

Believing the Disguise

Though narcissists project an air of independence, the reality is that they can't survive without a circle of admirers. For this reason, many narcissistic adults choose careers that will provide them with just such an audience. But in children and adults alike, the family is also expected to cater to the narcissist's ego. These demands are often made in disguise, delivered in ways that preserve the narcissist's illusion of autonomy. For example, a narcissistic parent may be very emotionally present when things are not going so well for them at work. The minute their career is on the upswing, they vanish from family life. When times are tough, the narcissist has a "good reason" for being emotionally needy or demanding.

Fearing Disapproval

There's nothing a narcissist hates more than humiliation. A spouse, child, or parent that does anything less than praise the narcissist may find themselves shunned, ignored, or neglected. As such, the family starts to fear the narcissist's disapproval. This can lead to parents funding extracurriculars that they can't afford, spouses attending functions that they hate, and children declaring majors in college that don't match their talents or interests.

Acceptance of Denial

Denial is one of the narcissist's most powerful and effective defenses. The spouses of narcissists, in particular, often find themselves expected to support and maintain the narcissist's lies, especially in public. Families will start to engage in a culture of denial themselves. Tantrums or abusive outbursts are simply ignored. Individual family members will start to hide or deny their hurt feelings when the narcissist behaves coldly or cruelly.

Effective Deception

Families headed by narcissistic parents can develop entire narcissistic cultures. They may teach their children that the family is special or that they don't have to do things the way that other families do them. These fantasies justify the family living outside the rules of normal society. What it also does is make it extremely hard for anyone to leave, as it becomes increasingly difficult and uncomfortable to interact with people outside the family.

Using Displacement

Slowly but surely, rules that apply to everyone else in the family seem to stop applying to the narcissist. This means that any negative feelings, such as annoyance, frustration, or aggravation, must find a new target if they are to be expressed at all. This can cause an excess of resentment and conflict that destroys the rest of the family, leaving the narcissist unscathed at the center of the chaos. Families learn to displace their anger at the narcissist onto other situations or even other people. Of course, this does nothing to resolve the anger and often leads to conflicts that are both unnecessary and permanently damaging.

Accepting Distortion

All personality disorders are founded on a skewed perception of reality. Families with narcissistic members often start to accept narcissistic distortions as their own personal, or even objective, realities. This, more than anything else, is what causes the family to start accepting and even protecting the narcissist's behaviors. This not only reinforces the narcissist's disorder, but it also makes it increasingly difficult for other members of the family to break free of the toxic dynamic. Even when they do recognize the narcissistic patterns that rule the family, people often feel guilty about the role they played in reinforcing them, which then prevents them from taking healthy steps to correct or remove themselves from the situation. This is especially true for parents who often feel responsible for a child's narcissistic behaviors. In an attempt to overcompensate for what they believe to have been a mistake on their part, they often make the situation much worse.

But guilt won't help you, your child, or your family. If you notice narcissistic behaviors in your child, it's helpful to take a look at the greater family dynamic. If your co-parent is narcissistic or alcoholic, this may call for more intense professional intervention and may be the source of your child's narcissistic traits. If you and/or your child have been in an abusive situation in the past, your child's narcissism could also have developed as a way to cope with that kind of home environment. In less extreme cases, any time a child internalizes the idea that love is conditional puts them at risk for narcissism. Examine your and your co-parent's parenting styles. And going forward, always show your child that you love them and that their behavior will not cause that love to be withdrawn.

It can be especially distressing for a parent with a narcissistic spouse to see those same traits appearing in their children. Though this can often trigger feelings of guilt or responsibility, remember that when you first married your spouse, you probably didn't realize that they had NPD. Don't blame yourself, and don't let yourself believe that it's too late for your child. If your spouse is narcissistic, your child's narcissistic behaviors may not have anything to do with their temperament or your parenting style. All children mimic their parents' behaviors, both good and bad. If they have a narcissistic parent, then they are bound to mimic narcissistic behaviors. The most effective way to combat this kind of mimicry is to teach your child empathy and make it clear how those behaviors make other people feel.

Many adults with NPD grew up in healthy, loving homes. There is increasing evidence that narcissistic personality disorder has a biological or genetic component, one whose influence cannot be ignored. Narcissism tends to run in families. It should also be mentioned that parents aren't the only family members from whom children can learn narcissistic behaviors. Narcissistic older siblings, grandparents, or even extended family members can all inadvertently pass narcissistic behaviors on to your child (Narcissist Abuse Support, 2019).

Rather than inadvertently enabling your child's narcissism, there are healthy steps you can take to correct and confront the narcissistic behaviors in your child (Narcissist Abuse Support, 2019):

Learn Coping Skills

Teach yourself and other members of the family healthy coping methods for dealing with the narcissistic child's behaviors. Teaching other children how to cope with their sibling will help to relieve their anxiety and fear. The narcissist often demands so much attention from their parents that their siblings feel neglected or ignored. Make sure that you are distributing your attention equally to all your children and that strategies for managing your child's narcissism don't inadvertently cause the family dynamics to revolve around them.

Set Boundaries

The earlier your child learns to accept the word "no," the happier and healthier they will be. Don't permit behaviors that disrupt the family. Instead, create rules that have clear consequences when broken. Make sure that your child understands the household rules and what will happen if they defy those rules. Make sure that whatever consequences you set are enforceable for both you and your co-parent.

Avoid Drama

Don't reward narcissistic behaviors with attention, even if it means physically leaving the situation for a moment or two. Remember, narcissists thrive off all kinds of attention, whether it's positive or negative.

Watch for Crumbs

Crumbs are small moments when the child pretends that they have overcome their narcissistic behaviors, often as an attempt to get something from you. Let go of the idea that if you just love your child enough, their "old self" will appear, and you can all go back to normal. Instead, focus on developing a happy and healthy "future self" for your child.

Learn to Live with Uncertainty

All parents worry about the safety and happiness of their children. This worry only increases when you know or suspect that your child has some kind of behavioral problem. But don't allow these fears to cause you to become smothering or overprotective. Narcissists are master manipulators, and a narcissistic child will learn to use your fear for their safety or well-being as a manipulative tool if you allow them to.

Don't Diagnose

Even if you're working together with a professional, avoid telling your child that they are a narcissist. This can cause the child to get stuck on the diagnosis and prevent them from reflecting clearly on their own behavior. They can also become obsessed with proving that there's "nothing wrong" with them or even trying to prove that *you* are the one with the problem.

Don't Argue

Arguing puts all people on the defensive, and with narcissists, this is doubly true. Arguing with your child will just make them more rigid and make them cling even more tightly to their defenses.

Focus on Choices

Let your child know that they can choose how they behave in any situation. Provide them with alternative places to channel their energy. Remember also that *you* have choices. Remind both yourself and your child that you are not obligated to accept behaviors that are destructive or hurtful.

Set Limits

Narcissists tend to disrupt a family dynamic slowly. Little by little, they demand more and more attention and loyalty. At the same time, their retaliations become more and more severe. Perhaps they start hurling insults, violate the family rules, or start manipulating other members of the family to get what they want. Don't allow this to happen. Always enforce the consequences for stepping over your or the family's boundaries.

Get Help

True narcissism is a very serious disorder, one that you shouldn't expect yourself to handle alone. Reaching out to friends, professionals, and counselors will give you the support and guidance you need to effectively manage your child's behaviors.

Monitor Conversations

Pay attention to conversations that your child is having at home, either with you or with other people. If your child tends to monopolize conversations, insist that they spend more time listening to others.

Ask Them to Contribute

Make sure that your child understands that everyone must contribute equally to the well-being of the household. Distribute chores equally, remind them to be considerate of other people's feelings, and make sure that they are not getting a disproportionate amount of attention.

Never Get Violent

It should go without saying that violence against children is abusive and never an acceptable way to parent. Though extremely narcissistic children can make you want to tear your (or their) hair out, remember that their behaviors are rooted in an extremely fragile self-esteem. Discipline firmly and consistently, but never show any kind of aggression toward your child.

The goal of early intervention for narcissistic children is to prevent them from growing into adults with full-blown narcissistic personality disorder. Remember that your narcissistic child will grow up to have a career and family of their own. If their narcissism remains unchecked, they may even go on to become a narcissistic parent.

While it's never too late to intervene in a narcissist's life, a teenager or young adult that's spent most of their life manipulating you and getting their way is going to be much more difficult to manage than a child who is still in the early stages of development. Narcissists can become extremely aggressive when someone they are used to pushing around starts setting boundaries. You cannot heal yourself or your family with an abusive person in your household. This late in life, the child's narcissistic tendencies are unlikely to go away, but they can still be managed, and a full-blown personality disorder can still be avoided.

Many spouses who end up in abusive marriages with narcissists often blame the narcissist's parents for not warning them or intervening to help them. The reason this never happens is that too many parents of narcissistic children hope that somehow their child's spouse will "fix" or "save" them. Frustrated parents may feel relieved when their narcissistic child gets married, feeling like the new spouse can share some of the burdens of managing the narcissist's abuse. None of these scenarios, of course, turn out to be true.

The Narcissistic Sibling

Growing up with a narcissistic sibling can, in many ways, be just as painful or damaging as growing up with a narcissistic parent. The sibling relationship is an intimate one, and you have probably seen the best and worst of your sibling while they were growing up. You may even feel guilty for not suspecting your sibling of having narcissism, despite the obvious warning signs.

For siblings, however, the diagnosis is much less important than the behaviors. If it helps, you can use the label as a way to name behaviors or dynamics that may have been difficult to articulate before. Understanding what motivates a narcissistic sibling can empower you to heal from the negative effects their behavior may have had on you as a child or even now as an adult. Knowledge about how the disorder disrupts family dynamics will help you to make beneficial decisions for yourself and your family moving forward.

Confronting the reality of a narcissistic sibling can be challenging because it also forces you to take a look at your own role in the toxic family dynamic. If one of your siblings is narcissistic, there's a good chance that one or both of your parents also had NPD. Children of narcissistic parents are also extremely likely to date or marry narcissists in the future. Learning about the role that narcissism played in your childhood will free you from seeing its influence in your own family in the future.

Your sibling may or may not have a diagnosis of NPD now. But as a child, it's unlikely that they received any kind of diagnosis or professional intervention. Until very recently, narcissism was understood as something that only appeared in adults. Psychologists in the 1980s began studying the ways that narcissism develops in childhood. Even then, it wasn't seen as something that could be prevented or treated.

Today, there is still much research to be done on how and why narcissism appears in children. What we do know is how to recognize some of the more obvious warning signs and how to treat them. In the past, however, your parents may not have had access to this kind of education or support. While it can be tempting for the siblings of narcissistic children to blame their parents, these kinds of feelings can prevent you from healing and moving forward from the narcissist's damage.

A narcissistic sibling will (Narcissist Abuse Support, 2019a):

- believe that they are more important than you and that they deserve to be recognized as such by other family members. Were there any jokes in the family about how your sibling was prettier or smarter than you?
- feel entitled to your parents' attention and special treatment. As adults, they feel entitled to your money and find ways to parasitically live off of you.
- be unable and unwilling to recognize your needs. This lack of empathy can be most hurtful when they fail to see how their behavior has hurt you. They resent having to listen to stories about your struggles, but they will insist that you listen to theirs. The same is true of your successes or achievements. They will become resentful and angry when you try to share the good things in your life but insist on telling you all about their own successes and victories.

- exaggerate their achievements and talents. What were exaggerations in childhood can quickly snowball into all-out lies in adolescence and adulthood. They may get angry when you try to ask for more details or fact check the stories they tell you. They may also tell lies about you to other members of the family. These lies may be designed to hurt your reputation or your status within the family.

- constantly tell you or your parents how great they are. This excessive need for admiration can be exhausting for everyone involved. Was your sibling extremely boastful or even pretentious as a child?

- be extremely envious of you. They may also speak about you very differently to people within the family vs. outsiders. If your sibling is constantly putting you down or telling other members of the family that you envy them but then sings your praises in public, beware. This is often a gimmick to make themselves look like a supportive and loving sibling.

- feel entitled to your parents' attention. They may monopolize conversations with you and other family members. They may constantly boast about their achievements or tell tales of their woes to gain sympathy from others. If they have the money, they may shower you or other family members with gifts to demonstrate just how caring and generous they are. No matter how they behave, it always seems to make them the center of attention.

- take advantage of you and other members of the family. If you have something they want, they will find a way to get it. More often than not, they do this with charm, so it can be very difficult to spot until it's too late.

- play whatever role they need to play to get what they want. A very common narcissistic mask is that of the victim. This is often used when they want attention from one or both parents. Another common mask is the "perfect" child. This can be very confusing for siblings of narcissists because they tend to see both the face that is presented to the parents and the face the narcissist wears when their parents aren't around.

- sabotage you and other members of the family. They may try something overt, like trying to have you taken out of the family will, or covert, like criticizing your choice of major in college. Either way, these behaviors are done with the goal of alienating you from the rest of the family.

- triangulate. This is what happens when one person pits two other people against each other.

Narcissists do this to prevent the family from uniting against them. For example, the narcissist may tell you something hurtful that another sibling "said." But unbeknownst to you, they're telling the other sibling lies about hurtful things that you "said," too. This keeps everyone else in the family embroiled in constant conflict, leaving them the only peaceful one at the center of all the chaos. Triangulation can be extremely psychologically damaging and makes it difficult to know who to trust. This is a common manipulation tactic employed by narcissistic parents, as well.

If you're unsure whether your sibling is narcissistic, there are a few questions you can ask yourself.

Do I enjoy being around them?

If the answer is no, then you know there's something amiss in your relationship. Children rarely enjoy spending time with a narcissistic sibling. Being around them can be exhausting, whether it's one-on-one or together with other family members. Feelings of anxiety or depression before you see them are another big indicator that something is wrong. Non-narcissistic siblings often ignore these warning signs out of a sense of obligation to be with their siblings or keep the family peace.

Is it hard to talk to them?

Conversations with narcissists often feel overwhelming or confusing. They also tend to be relatively one-sided. Narcissists will often talk "at" you without allowing you to get a word in edgewise. They may also have a tendency to bring up painful or humiliating memories from the past in conversations with other people. If you feel like your conversations always descend into some form of the blame-game, this is another sign that something is wrong in your relationship.

Am I always the loser in any argument?

Do you never seem able to win any fight, even when you're clearly right? Narcissistic siblings always need to win, and that means that you must always lose. Evidence to support your arguments has no effect. They will put you down or even deny your achievements. If it somehow happens that you find yourself in the family spotlight, they will dig up painful or humiliating memories from the past to tarnish your image. Whenever you receive praise, they are quick to undermine it. This often makes siblings of narcissists feel like they have to compete for their parents' attention, which can either cause them to develop narcissistic tendencies of their own or major depression later in life.

Are they able (or unable) to take responsibility for their actions?

A narcissistic sibling never seems to be at fault. This trait often begins very early in childhood and is often a trait that siblings see before parents or other family members. Did your sisters always blame you for things that she did? Would your brother intentionally break rules or play tricks and then tell your parents you did it? As an adult, does your sibling continue to blame you for their own choices? Narcissistic siblings never learn that it's OK to make mistakes. Instead, they spend their entire lives shifting the blame or the consequences of their actions onto their siblings or other family members.

Do they ask me to lie for them or keep their secrets?

This is another trait that often starts very early in childhood. The siblings of narcissists often spend a great deal of their time and energy covering things up or cleaning up after the narcissist. If they do reveal one of the narcissist's secrets, the retaliation can be terrible. Many narcissistic siblings even resort to physical or verbal abuse of their siblings in order to keep them compliant in their games.

Do we have an ongoing rivalry?

Narcissists are always in competition with their siblings. Many families, especially dysfunctional ones, can sometimes encourage sibling rivalries in order to make the children smarter or stronger. Some families will even intentionally place their children on rival sports teams to increase the competitive spirit. This can be an incredibly painful way to grow up and can drive siblings apart from a very young age.

Do I feel like the crazy sibling?

To make themselves look better, narcissists will often tell stories to other members of the family, designed to make you look crazy or unstable. This can be overt, such as saying outright nasty things about you to other people, or covert, like baiting you into an argument that they know will make you look bad. Over time, this tactic can indeed lead to psychological problems in their siblings, which only makes it more difficult to defend against the narcissist's manipulations.

Do they respect my boundaries?

Narcissistic siblings tend to have terrible boundaries because they feel entitled to your time, energy, or things. This often begins in early childhood, especially with siblings who share a bedroom. For example, imagine that your parents take you to the store and tell you each to pick out a cupcake for dessert. Perhaps you picked chocolate, and they picked vanilla. Then, after dinner, your sibling throws a tantrum, saying that they changed their mind and now they want chocolate. Your parents ask you to be a good sibling and let your brother or sister have the chocolate cupcake. This might seem innocent, but it teaches the narcissistic sibling that they can have anything they want from you.

Have they betrayed my confidence or trust?

Betrayal stings, and between siblings, it can take years to get over. But narcissistic siblings have a tendency to string up multiple betrayals throughout the course of a lifetime. The reason for this is that they are very good at worming their way back into your life and often back into your trust. After most people betray you, you distance yourself from them and never let it happen again. Narcissists are so manipulative that even the most vigilant of people find themselves starting to forgive their past indiscretions. Family members are the most vulnerable to this kind of manipulation, as they have the closest personal relationship with the narcissist. Often they will make a show of remorse or guilt for what they've done to you in the past. And then, before you even realize what's happening, they've betrayed you again. Worse, they tend to disappear after the betrayal or even blame you for it.

Think back to a time that your sibling betrayed you. How did you feel? Did you eventually allow them back into your trust? Being betrayed over and over can often make siblings of narcissists feel like there's something wrong with them. You may feel stupid or take out your frustration on yourself or other family members rather than on the narcissist. Remember that a betrayal is never your fault. Going forward, be as cautious as you can with your narcissistic sibling, and don't blame yourself if they manage to betray you again.

If you do suspect that your sibling is a narcissist, there a few steps you can take to protect yourself from their behaviors in the future (Narcissist Abuse Support, 2019a):

Do Not Confront Them

Feel free to tell other members of the family your suspicions. But don't try to tell your sibling that you think they're a narcissist. First, they will probably not listen to or believe you. It is more likely that they will also try to retaliate against what they will inevitably see as an insult. If they think you're about to get out from under their control, they start telling lies or spreading harmful rumors about you in order to discredit you before you can talk to anyone else.

Listen To Yourself

You are not obligated to have your sibling in your life. Ask yourself what kinds of behaviors you are willing to allow from your siblings and what you will do if they treat you in ways that are unacceptable. If something feels wrong, then listen to and honor your own feelings.

Set Good Boundaries

If you have a narcissistic sibling, chances are good that you never learned how to set good boundaries. Setting good boundaries means clearly telling the other person what behavior (or behaviors) you can no longer accept from them. Then, make it clear that there will be consequences if they violate that boundary. Make sure that the consequences you set are both specific and enforceable. Otherwise, when they inevitably push the boundary, all you're telling them is that there's nothing you can do about it. It's also important to remember that a boundary is only a boundary once it's clearly communicated to the other person. No one should have to read your mind. It's your responsibility to make it clear what you can and cannot accept, and if they violate those boundaries, then the other person is responsible for handling the consequences of that violation.

Boundaries are extremely difficult for all kinds of people, so do not feel bad about yourself if you struggle with them. Many siblings of narcissists also tend to develop codependent tendencies, which can make boundary work even more difficult. If you feel intimidated or confused, try practicing with a friend or a therapist before having the conversation with your sibling.

Protecting and Empowering the Family Unit

Recognizing and managing narcissism isn't something that one person can do alone. A narcissist can't always recognize or admit that they have a problem. This is especially true in children who are still developing their identity and sense of self in relation to the world. This means that the narcissist themself cannot actively participate in the management or treatment of their own disorder.

Narcissism is also a disorder that feeds off of dysfunctional relationship dynamics. Narcissists actively seek out other people that they can bend to their own will, derive attention and admiration from, and blame or punish for their negative feelings. You may be able to successfully manage your child's narcissism when you're one-on-one with them, but the less able they are to control you, the more actively they will seek to disrupt and manipulate other members of the family. This can cause you and the rest of the family to slip into a dysfunctional dynamic with the narcissist, no matter how vigilant you may be.

In order to make a successful intervention with a narcissistic child, everyone in the home must be on the same page. You and your co-parent should both have an understanding of NPD as a disorder, which symptoms your child is exhibiting, and how to manage those symptoms when they arise. If you and your co-parent are not in clear communication with each other, this makes it very easy for the narcissist to tell lies, pit you both against each other, and otherwise wreak havoc in the household.

First and foremost, if you suspect one or more of your children is showing warning signs of NPD, try to take an honest look at the family dynamic and ask yourself these questions (Nair, 2018):

- Has the child been pampered or made to feel special?
- Are you overdependent on or overprotective of the child?
- Have you been absent, physically or emotionally, from the child's upbringing?

- Do you often criticize the child?
- Do other members of the family display narcissistic traits, including grandparents, uncles, or aunts? Is only one child displaying narcissistic traits, or do you suspect multiple siblings of developing NPD?
- Is your child adopted?
- Have you and/or your child been in an abusive home in the past?
- Are you divorced from the child's other parent?
- Did anyone in your childhood home have narcissistic traits?
- Is your child hypersensitive?
- Does your spouse and/or the child's co-parent have narcissistic traits?

Asking yourself these questions can give you some idea of where the child's narcissism may be coming from and therefore give you guidance as to the best way to intervene on the child's behalf.

The next step is to sit down with your co-parent, and possibly with the child's siblings if they are old enough, and determine which symptoms the narcissistic child is displaying. Do they show:

- a sense of entitlement?
- a lack of empathy?
- beliefs that they have unlimited power or special abilities?

- high levels of self-importance?
- gaze aversion or an obvious discomfort with eye contact?
- high expectations of respect and adoration?
- a sense of superiority?
- separation anxiety?
- a tendency to blame others for their bad behaviors?
- a tendency to exaggerate or outright lie about their achievements?
- a willingness to exploit others?
- a selfish or haughty attitude?
- envy towards others?
- a sense of enjoyment in pathological games?
- opportunistic behaviors?
- a strange sense of formality, even in close relationships?
- a high sensitivity to criticism?

Getting a clear idea of the symptoms that need to be addressed will not only give you and other members of the family a clear idea of what you're dealing with, but it will help you to determine whether or not professional intervention is necessary. If you do believe that it's time to contact a professional, make sure that you and your co-parent are both in agreement that you believe your child is displaying signs of narcissistic personality disorder. Remember that any therapist, even one who specializes in personality disorders, will try to rule out other possibilities before giving your child a definitive diagnosis. Physical tests are not an uncommon part of the diagnostic process, including the ordering of brain scans to detect any potential neurological causes for your child's behavior. For this reason, it's typically safer to contact a therapist rather than the child's pediatrician about behavioral concerns. While a medical doctor will rarely order a psychiatric evaluation, a psychologist will typically order any physical tests that they deem necessary. Knowing this can give you and your co-parent relative peace of mind if you do decide to take your child in for professional evaluation. Since therapists are very hesitant to diagnose young children with narcissism, the chances of your child being misdiagnosed are relatively unlikely. It's also important that both you and your co-parent are in regular contact with your child's therapist so that both of you are getting the exact same information.

If your child is a teenager, their narcissism may have already created other complications, including relationship troubles with friends or other members of the family. If you are worried about your child's ability to make friends or their social skills, this is also something to mention to your therapist. Additional professional intervention may be required if your child is developing a dependence on drugs or alcohol.

Your co-parent is probably not the only person who is affected by your child's narcissism. If the child has siblings or close relationships with other members of the family, those people should be included in the intervention if at all possible or appropriate. Older siblings, grandparents, and extended family members can all act as a grounding influence on the child. They can also give you and your co-parent much needed support.

Siblings, especially younger ones, are particularly vulnerable to narcissistic attacks and manipulations. Not only do they have a dysfunctional relationship with the narcissist, but the narcissist's destructive traits have most likely damaged their relationship with other members of the family. Narcissists disrupt normal, nurturing family dynamics, and that prevents the siblings of the narcissist from getting the love and support they need growing up. Narcissists are often envious of their siblings and tend to control the family dynamic in a way that benefits them at their sibling(s)' expense (Bash, 2017).

Siblings are often the first people to see and experience the damaging effects of emerging narcissism. They often don't realize how dangerous their sibling can be until the damage has already been done. Worse, the narcissist typically has a great deal of control over the family dynamic, and that includes their parents' perceptions of the relationship between siblings. If the narcissist suspects that the sibling is going to say something to their parents, they will often intervene to make the sibling look crazy, spoiled, or attention-seeking. They can also play games with their siblings, punishing them for telling the narcissist's secrets, doing something better than the narcissist, or even simply getting positive attention from their parents (Hammond, 2018).

All of this can cause narcissistic siblings to live in the family shadows. They often live in fear of their narcissistic sibling's wrath, and as such, avoid stepping into the spotlight as much as possible. Many grow up with low self-esteem or develop codependent behaviors later in life because they spend their childhoods catering to the narcissistic sibling's needs and not their own. They may begin to compete with the narcissist for their parents' attention or even develop narcissistic traits of their own. If you are unsure about whether or not your child displays any narcissistic symptoms, the people who will know the real answer are the narcissist's siblings.

As the popular awareness of NPD increases, more and more siblings of people with narcissistic personality disorder are starting to speak out about their experiences growing up. This has led psychologists to understand that narcissistic traits emerge much earlier in life than was previously thought. Children can indeed express pathological levels of envy, devaluation, and lack of empathy towards others, levels that go beyond normal childhood narcissism. While exploitative behaviors and lack of empathy may compromise their relationships at school, their siblings have little recourse or protection from their devaluations (Bridges to Recovery, 2020).

Narcissistic behaviors can create dynamics within a family unit that are both painful and profoundly disorienting for their siblings. The experience of having a sibling with NPD is uniquely traumatizing, as siblings often become the direct or indirect victims of the narcissist's attempts to preserve their own distorted view of themselves. The narcissist tends to mold the behavior of the family around their needs (and their needs only), leaving the emotional needs of the sibling largely unattended. The sibling's ability to develop in an emotionally healthy way is, therefore, doubly compromised, both by the narcissistic sibling's abuse and the inevitable parental neglect.

Narcissistic children often develop an insatiable need for attention and a strong sense of entitlement. In order to satisfy these needs, they start to seek out other people from which they can exact the attention and adoration that they need to maintain their sense of superiority. In children, the nearest available person is typically their siblings, even before their parents. The stronger the narcissist's traits become, the more adulation, compliments, and admiration they start to demand from their siblings. And the more their dysfunctional worldview is supported, the more desperate their tactics for exacting this kind of tribute become.

Siblings make an easy target for narcissists because of their powerlessness and vulnerability within the family hierarchy. Some narcissists can become outright abusive toward their siblings, punishing them with verbal abuse like ridiculing or belittling in order to establish the narcissist's superiority. This cruelty is often hidden from parents, especially in young children. The constant demands for attention and punishments for not giving it often cause the narcissist's sibling to believe that they are personally responsible for the narcissist's happiness.

In some cases, narcissists can even become physically or sexually abusive toward their siblings (Hammond, 2018).

The trauma of growing up with a narcissistic sibling can be complex, as it involves multiple levels of pain and psychological disruption. Siblings are often denied the positive attention and nurturing they need from their parents at a critical time in their development. Siblings often grow up to be codependent, which not only prevents them from caring for their own needs in future relationships but predisposes them to have romantic partnerships or even marry someone with NPD later in life. The siblings of narcissists are also at high risk for drug and alcohol abuse. These problems often develop alongside their sibling's narcissism, but their emotional turmoil is often overshadowed by the narcissist's drama.

If your narcissistic child has siblings, then their recovery is another crucial part of the narcissistic intervention. Support for a narcissistic child can sometimes be yet another way in which the narcissist's siblings are taught to deny their own needs and feelings for the sake of the narcissist's well-being. If you determine that your narcissistic child needs professional help, then you can almost guarantee that your other children also need professional guidance in recovering from whatever damage the narcissist has already caused. You can ask the same therapist that evaluates your narcissistic child what they recommend as therapy options for your other children. Depending on the age of your other children and the severity of the narcissist's symptoms, the therapist may recommend individual psychotherapy, refer you to support groups for siblings of narcissists, or suggest a combination of both. These will help your other children to establish healthy coping behaviors and recover their psychological wellness. A therapist can also give your children strategies for guarding themselves against future traumatic interactions with their sibling. It also widens your own network of support in managing your narcissistic child's disruptive behaviors (Bridges to Recovery, 2020).

Depending on your child's symptoms, your therapist may recommend psychoanalytic therapy. This will involve both one-on-one sessions between a professional and your child, as well as counseling for you and your co-parent. Some therapists recommend family therapy as the appropriate intervention, which would involve the entire household going to therapy together as a group. Cognitive behavior treatment is a third option that would involve intense, one-on-one work between your child and a professional. If this is the recommended course of treatment, ask your child's therapist if there's anything you can do at home to reinforce what they are learning or working on in therapy.

Narcissists thrive on secrets, lies, and triangulation. Therefore, the more unified the family is against the narcissist, the more effective the intervention will be. If everyone in the family is aware of the behaviors, the narcissist will be less able to get away with bullying, lying, or manipulating. Everyone must be committed to giving the narcissist the same treatment and holding them to the same standards of accountability as everyone else in the family.

You and your co-parent should also be on the same page in terms of consequences. If and when the narcissistic child does violate the household rules, they must get the same response from both parents. If one parent is aggressive or enabling, this will only worsen the child's narcissistic tendencies.

As much as you can, create clear systems of rules and behavior that everyone in the house follows. Something visible and trackable, such as a posted schedule for chores or homework, can help the narcissist to internalize the balance of responsibility within the family dynamic and help the rest of the family to keep the narcissist accountable. A similar model can be used to help your child practice their listening skills. Family activities that allow one person to speak at a time, such as going around the table at dinner and saying what you're thankful for, limits the narcissist's ability to monopolize conversations.

Above all, make sure that the intervention remains an intervention, not a punishment. Remember that narcissism is deeply rooted in a low sense of self-worth. If the child feels targeted or singled out, this will only serve to shatter an already fragile self-esteem. Demonstrate your love to the child as often as you can. Teach them how to recognize empathy and kindness within themselves. Teach them that everyone has unique strengths, and encourage them to find those strengths in themselves and in other people. The earlier you and your family make this kind of intervention, the happier and healthier your child will grow up to be.

Chapter 5:

Helping Your Child

It can be very difficult to intervene once a child has started to show signs of narcissism. The easiest way to manage narcissistic personality disorder is to prevent it from developing in the first place.

The first and most obvious way to prevent narcissism is to simply love your children. Show them that love is unwavering and unconditional, even when they fail or behave badly. One of the greatest gifts a parent can give a child is to show them that you can recognize their failings and still love them. True love, however, is not performance based. Try not to withhold love as a punishment for underachieving or teach your children that they need to compete for your affection. The more comfortable you are at recognizing and accepting your child's flaws (which they do have), the better able you will be to love them exactly for who they are. No one is perfect, and no child will grow up to be perfect. Once you've accepted this truth, you can stop loving who your child *could* or *should* be and start loving your child for who they are.

That being said, most parents don't have to be taught to love their children. Even the most loving households can still produce narcissists. This is because parents don't always realize the kinds of unconscious messages that they send their children with certain parenting styles or techniques. Many people rely on their own parents as an example of what to do (or not do) when raising children. All children and childhoods are different. Your child may not have the same needs that you or your siblings did growing up. Your child is also growing up in a very different world from the one that you grew up in, and as such, the challenges they experience and messages they receive in the outside world may cause them to view the world very differently from the way you did at their age.

Recent studies of narcissism have been increasingly focused on its origins in early childhood. Since factors like biology or random events are impossible to control, the hope is that, by understanding which parenting styles contribute to the development of NPD, the condition can be greatly minimized in the general population. Recently, the National Academy of Sciences published a study that found parents who overvalue their children were more likely to raise narcissists than other kinds of parents. The study found that parents of narcissistic children were more likely to answer affirmatively to statements like "my child is more special than other children" or "my child deserves something extra in life." Brad Bushman, coauthor of the study, summarized these findings by saying that when parents tell their children they are special, they believe it. Far from bolstering their self-esteem, this belief can both damage their development and have negative consequences for the people around them (Hamaker, 2017).

It's not difficult to understand why it's problematic for a child to believe they're better than everyone else. More often than not, this belief begins with their parents. Children who hear their parents brag about them all the time will inevitably believe all the good things their parents say about them. Why wouldn't they?

Yet, raising your child to be "extra-special" doesn't necessarily make you a bad parent. In fact, during the 1990s, this is what parents were recommended to do. We now know how damaging such a parenting style can be, but there's still a lot in popular culture and parenting advice that steers well-meaning parents in this direction (Hamaker, 2017).

The question, then, is how to raise your child to have strong self-esteem without slipping into overpraising or overvaluing language. Here are a few simple strategies that you and your co-parent can add to your parenting styles to help prevent the development of narcissism and other personality disorders in your children.

Praise Clearly and Concisely

Vague statements of praise like "You're so great!" can be interpreted in many different ways, especially by an insecure child. The more specific you are with your praise, the more clear it is to the child what exactly is being recognized. "I'm proud of you for working so hard at this!" or "I'm so impressed that you still tried your best, even though you don't like that class" are examples of praise that tell the child it's their efforts and actions that are being recognized, not their overall character.

Praise is feedback, just as much as criticism. The more specific the praise, the more clearly you understand what you've done well. The more clearly you understand what you've done well, the more likely you are to do it again in the future. Specific praise is also much more meaningful than general or vague statements. When we praise specific actions or behaviors, we're also telling our children that we've been paying attention to them and their lives.

Praise the Present

"You did a great job cleaning your room today" is much better than "You're always so helpful around the house!" Again, this makes it clear that the thing being praised is the child's specific action or accomplishment. Words like "always" and "never" can be internalized by the child as evaluative statements. They give the action that's being praised much greater significance than it probably deserves. Generalizations also devalue individual achievements. After all, if you "always" do a good job, then doing a good job isn't something special. When you anchor your compliments in the present moment, it gives your child the opportunity to feel like they've done something special and prompts them to reflect on what they did "today" that was so extraordinary. This, in turn, motivates them to rise to similar standards in the future for their own sake, and not because their self-worth is hanging in the balance.

Praise Sparingly

Believe it or not, children don't need a continuous stream of praise to feel good about themselves. On the contrary, this can hinder their ability to develop an innate sense of self-worth. Of course, it's perfectly OK to recognize your child's achievements and talents. Too much praise can create a craving for it. It sends the message to the child that when they're not being praised, something is wrong. If you go out of your way to compliment every effort they make, they can start to believe that they're somehow special or even better than other people who aren't praised as often. Overpraising can also lessen the emotional impact of your attention. Rather than feeling recognized or appreciated, the child comes to expect that level of appreciation all the time. However, be wary of praising too little, as this can damage your child's self-esteem or make them feel like they have to earn your affection.

Praise What is Extraordinary

Praising and celebrating every single thing a child does will raise them to expect a high level of attention all the time. Never praising or acknowledging your child's accomplishments can damage their self-esteem. To strike a good balance, praise what is worthy of praising. When your child accomplishes something you know was difficult or makes an extraordinary effort to push themselves, let them know that you're proud of the work that they do. Praising their efforts and actions rather than praising *them* helps them to understand the connection between hard work and positive outcomes. It also helps them to recognize that they are not inherently better or worse than anyone else.

Determining what is "worthy" of praise may seem like a cold and evaluative way to look at your child. But if you try it, you'll probably find the opposite to be true. When you stop praising every move your child makes and start thinking about what you're praising and why, you'll probably find yourself paying closer attention to your child's actual life. In reality, not everything your child does is worth celebrating. There are probably many ways in which your child *does* do things that astonish and genuinely impress you. If you save your praise for these moments, your words feel more genuine and therefore be more appreciated. You'll also find that you stop praising the achievements (e.g., the good grades) and start praising the work your child did to achieve them (e.g., going for extra help after school).

Teach the Golden Rule

"Do unto others as you would have them do unto you." Teaching this rule to your children will help them to learn empathy for others. Using this rule to check their motivations and actions will help them to practice thinking about what life might be like for other people and what kind of effects their actions may have on others' well-being.

This is especially important for children growing up in today's individualist, highly-digitized culture. Not only are they unlikely to get empathetic messages or teachings from the culture at large, but it's also much more difficult to see the impact of their words and actions online. If you say something mean to another child at school, you'll see them burst into tears or turn red-faced with anger. If you say something hurtful online, chances are that you will never have to face the consequences of that communication. If children aren't actively prompted to think about how other people might feel, they may never learn to conceive of the people around them as having needs or feelings, too.

Model Empathy

The best way to teach empathy is to practice it yourself. Take as many opportunities as you can to explain to your children how other people are feeling, or ask them how they would feel in such a situation. This teaches our children to view the world from a compassionate rather than a competitive place. Reading is another great way to teach children empathy, as it encourages them to imagine and experience life from another person's perspective.

Combat Entitlement

Make sure there is always a balance between giving and contributing. As children get older, make sure there are clear expectations in terms of chores and general household rules of respect. Of course, there's nothing wrong with giving your children gifts or treats, but continuous gift-giving has the same effect as continuous praise—over time, your children will stop appreciating them and start expecting them.

Listen to Your Children

Narcissists expect you to do what they say when they say it. When your child is making demands, try to listen to what they're *really* saying. If your child is having a meltdown because they don't like the outfit you chose for them in the morning, what they might actually be saying is that they're overwhelmed or feeling sick; they may even be trying to let you know they're being bullied at school.

Don't Play the Rescuer

As difficult and painful as it can be, you must allow your children to experience failure. If they make a mistake, support them in recovering from it. If you are always there to clean up their messes, or worse, try to protect them from their failures, you can foster feelings of entitlement in your child and teach them that they are not accountable for their own actions. Allow your child to feel the consequences of their actions and only rescue them when your child is in real danger.

Give Attention Selectively

It's OK to let your child know that you have your own life. Encourage periods of reading, play, or study in which you and the child are engaged in your own activities. As a parent, you know that your life revolves around your child. If they can see that, then they will start to expect that level of attention from you and from everyone else.

Parent Consistently

Chaotic and abusive parenting styles can cause deep-seated feelings of insecurity in a child. If your child learns that they can't depend on you, then they start to believe that they can only depend on themselves. This can lead to both egocentric behavior and a suspicion of authority.

Enforce Consequences

If your child violates the household rules or boundaries, never let it slide. Only accept excuses in very rare and extraordinary circumstances. If you see your child violating the boundaries of others, make sure to teach them long-term relational skills, like asking them to apologize when they've said something hurtful or teaching them effective ways to handle bullies.

Call Out Narcissism

Don't actually call your child a narcissist. But don't hesitate to name or point out their symptoms such as saying, "Demanding more than your fair share is called 'entitlement'" or "Calling people names is aggressive." These are examples of ways you can help them to recognize the problems in their own behavior.

Teach Good Values

Teach your children to value character traits like honesty and kindness, either directly or indirectly. There's much in our culture that subliminally teaches our children that they must be tough or dominant. Pay attention to the kinds of people you praise or encourage your children to look up to. Who are you holding up to your children as role models, and why?

Don't Play the Blame Game

Don't allow your child to blame other people for their own bad behaviors. Even in situations when someone else was clearly at fault, teach your child coping skills. If your child gets in a fight at school, teach them how to stand up to bullies without resorting to violence. If your child made a comment that accidentally hurt someone's feelings, teach them ways to improve their social skills.

Build Your Child's Self-Esteem

Low self-esteem isn't just linked to narcissism. It's at the root of all personality disorders and many other psychological problems. Healthy self-esteem means believing that one has inherent value and worthiness, but not *more* value or worthiness than other people.

Teach Stress and Frustration Management

Protecting your child from adversity prevents them from developing the skills they need to overcome it. This certainly doesn't mean you should intentionally challenge your child or put them in harm's way. It does mean that when they inevitably experience the everyday challenges of life, you're there to teach them how to overcome those challenges. Teach them how to live with negative feelings like disappointment or frustration, rather than trying to insulate them from ever having those feelings.

Healthy Parenting Techniques for Narcissism Management and Prevention

Not all narcissistic symptoms present themselves in a severe or alarming way. There's quite a big difference between NPD and narcissistic traits. With so many examples of narcissism in our popular culture, from athletes to actors to political leaders, it can sometimes feel inevitable when your child starts mimicking the behaviors of these famous and influential figures. So how can you determine when your child's behaviors are normal, manageable, or subclinically narcissistic?

Determining the difference between normal childhood narcissism and concerning levels of narcissistic behavior is the biggest challenge parents face. If you have a normal 2-year-old, you will probably feel like they exemplify every symptom on the list of concerning behaviors. Most children either grow out of these behaviors or only engage in them during moments of stress or frustration. Many therapists insist that narcissism simply cannot be diagnosed in children under the age of 13 because until that age, it's almost impossible to differentiate it from normal childhood narcissism (*How to Deal with a Child with Narcissistic Personality Disorder*, 2019).

Recent studies have suggested that parenting styles are the biggest predictor of NPD, more than biological or other environmental factors (Dawson, 2015). This puts a lot of pressure on parents and can lead to feelings of shame or guilt if you do suspect your child is narcissistic. There is still substantial evidence to suggest that narcissism most likely has a biological component that exists alongside the conditions of childhood. If your child is not genetically predisposed and lives in a reasonably loving home, it's unlikely that they will grow up to develop NPD. Remember, there's a big difference between someone with pronounced narcissistic traits and someone with an outright personality disorder. Those with narcissistic traits, if they learn how to manage them, can grow up to live very healthy and successful lives. Not everything can be changed with parenting, but the right interventions can go a long way toward lessening the impact of problematic behaviors. And if your child is 18 or older, it's still never too late to change your interactions in ways that will benefit their development through adulthood. More importantly, narcissistic traits in adulthood can still be successfully managed without radical professional intervention.

When managing your child's narcissism, it can sometimes be helpful to focus on individual symptoms (Hammond, 2016):

Entitlement

Is your child entitled or simply exercising their autonomy? How do they respond when you ask them to do chores or hold them accountable for shirking their duties?

The easiest way to fight entitlement in your child is to just say "no." Don't worry—saying this word won't turn you into an authoritarian tyrant, nor will it crush your child's creative spirit. If your child is trying to set something on fire or steal extra sweets out of the cupboard, it's not only fine to say no, it's critically important. The earlier your child learns to accept that they can't have whatever they want, the less entitled they will feel or behave. Learning to hear the word "no" will also teach them to respect the rules and boundaries that they encounter from other people later in life.

Ego

Is your child super-confident, or do they believe that they are superior to others? How does their confidence affect other people in the household? A child with healthy self-esteem will not drain the emotional energy of the people around them.

A simple way to manage the size of your child's ego is to teach them basic manners. When you think of a "snobby" person, what's the first image that comes to mind? Most likely, it's an image of someone being rude to a waiter or refusing to eat a meal that doesn't cater to their special diet. Manners are the societal version of household or classroom rules. Being polite is how we show respect to other people, even strangers or professionals that we've never met. Rudeness is a signal to the world that you have no respect for others or believe that the rules of common society don't apply to you.

Empathy

Does your child lack empathy or social skills? Do they expect others to read their mind or cater to their feelings? How do they react to the news that something they said or did may have hurt someone else? Are they able to learn from conflict, or do they blame other people for their own negative feelings?

Though it may not seem obvious, frustration and stress management skills work hand-in-hand with building empathy. Children who aren't allowed to feel their own negative feelings have a difficult time recognizing them in other people. Children who aren't able to manage their negative feelings may start to lash out at other people. Teaching your child how to work through their negative feelings will increase their ability to recognize and care for people who are experiencing negative feelings of their own.

Demands

Does your child make unreasonable demands, or is there often a deeper reason for bad behavior? How do they respond when you explain why their demands cannot be met? Are they still throwing frequent tantrums beyond the age of five?

Saying "no" to your child isn't easy or enjoyable. Imagine that your child flies into a rage because her sister got something that she didn't. If you change your behavior in response to your child's tantrum, what you're teaching her is that if she wants something from you, all she has to do is fly into a rage, and you'll get it for her. The time to teach her that she can't have everything she wants isn't later on when she's calm: it's right then and there when she's throwing a tantrum. Staring down a storm of hurt and rage doesn't feel good, especially when it's in public. The more tantrums she gets away with, the more rages you can expect in the future.

Catering to a child's unrealistic demands might soothe them in the moment, but it doesn't help them in the long-run. NPD aside, catering to a child's rage doesn't provide them with healthy ways to cope with negative feelings like anger or disappointment. Nor will it teach them how to feel happy for the successes or fortunes of other people.

Victim Playing

When things go wrong, does your child always find a way to make someone else responsible? When they explain their side of the story, are they still able to take responsibility for their own actions? Are they able to engage with proactive solutions for dealing with bullies, institutional prejudices, and other external pressures?

Victim mentalities and behaviors often appear in people (children or adults) who feel they aren't getting enough love or support. The victim behavior isn't always a behavior—your child may genuinely feel like everyone and everything is working against them. If you notice these kinds of behaviors, try to determine where they're coming from. If your child is feeling unnoticed or unloved, where are those feelings coming from? What can you do to repair their damaged self-esteem? While you're doing work to set stricter rules and boundaries, don't forget to show your child the warmth and kindness they need to feel loved.

Attention-Seeking

All children crave attention from their parents. But how much is too much? Is your child satisfied with intermittent praise and quality time, or do they resort to negative attention when they aren't getting enough positive focus? It's normal for a 2-year-old to throw a tantrum to get attention—it's not normal for a 12-year-old.

All attention is not equal, especially when it comes to children. Too much of the wrong kind of attention and not enough of the right attention can both cause disturbances in your child's self-esteem and lead to narcissistic traits like entitlement or disregarding other people's feelings. The wrong kind of attention comes from parenting styles like overvaluing, overprotecting, or rescuing. The right kind of attention, of course, is true parental love, and a lack of it can look like parental absence (physical or emotional), coldness, or abuse. All of these parenting styles make a child feel small and unimportant. This might not be as intuitive with behaviors like pampering or rescuing, but think about these behaviors from the child's perspective. Though it may seem like you're protecting or saving your child from unpleasant feelings and dangerous situations, what you're actually teaching your child is that they're incompetent. Pampering subliminally sends the message to the child that they are incapable of solving their own problems or even feeling their own feelings. This makes them emotionally dependent on you and your approval in order to feel safe and worthy. Worse, it can cause them to overcompensate for feelings of smallness and insecurity by developing a grandiose persona or demanding whatever it is they want from you or other people (Frazier, 2015).

Strange though it might sound, a good remedy for attention-seeking behavior is to travel with your children. Whether you go to another country or the next town over, the important thing is to take your child somewhere new and different. It doesn't have to be expensive or extravagant. The point is to foster a sense of curiosity in your child and to show them that there's a big, wide world beyond their little social bubble.

Self-Esteem

Does your child have healthy self-esteem? If you aren't sure, simply ask your child if they believe they will be loved no matter what they do or say. If the answer to that question is anything but *yes*, it may be time to take active steps to improve your child's sense of self-worth.

Remember always that love and approval are two different things. Suspecting that your love is contingent upon your approval can be incredibly damaging to a child's self-esteem. Show them that you always love them, even when you're angry or disappointed with them. When your child becomes secure in the knowledge that your love won't be withdrawn, they can begin to relax and accept themselves for who they are.

The mythological story of Narcissus reminds us of what narcissistic personality disorder really is. At its core, narcissism is the experience of having too much self-love. Like Narcissus in the story, it's not real love. Instead, it's the constant need to find external approval for what the narcissist is feeling inside. Therefore, the most powerful intervention against narcissism a parent can make is to teach their child what true love looks and feels like.

Inherent or External?

Is your child's behavior becoming a consistent part of their personality? Or are they reacting to something in their environment? Acting out and misbehaving is a very common way for children to signal to the adults around them that something is wrong, something that they may not know how to articulate.

One very literal way to give your children the words they need to express themselves is to read to them. Reading won't just improve your child's vocabulary—it will also help to improve their empathy, teach them about the world, and sharpen their critical thinking skills. Stories are one of the oldest and most effective ways humans have to teach our children the emotional and interpersonal skills they need to function happily in society.

Bold or Bossy?

Does your child like to take charge and lead the group? Or are they bullying the other children around them? If other children are afraid of your child, then it's time to start teaching them better interpersonal skills.

It might be a headache at first, but if you see your child behaving like a tyrant, bring them along the next time you have errands to run. Letting your child see all the work you do every day to care for yourself and the family will give them a valuable lesson in responsibility. Though your child may not get it at first, insisting that they run errands with you is a way of insisting that they contribute to the general good of the household. If they are running your errands with you, then they will start to understand that your primary function in life isn't entertaining them. If they can start to feel like they're contributing to the daily operations of the family, then they can learn there's joy to be had in helping others.

Criticism

No one likes receiving negative feedback or criticism, especially not young children. But when you do have to criticize, does your child get upset, or do they emotionally fall apart? Do they become resentful or vengeful when you praise their siblings or other children around them?

Making an effort to change your parenting style and pulling back from overvaluing parenting habits will not only benefit your child, but it will also give you a clearer idea of the severity of your child's symptoms. If you believe that your child is perfect, special, and can do no wrong, then you are unlikely to recognize their narcissistic symptoms for what they really are. And if you truly believe your child is perfect and special, then you are unlikely to have gotten so far into this book.

But even well-meaning parents can inadvertently send damaging messages or create dysfunctional dynamics with their children. It may even be fair to say that it's "normal" for a family to have some kind of dysfunction! With narcissism awareness on the rise, it would be reasonable for the parents of a very healthy toddler to suspect their child may be developing NPD.

Whatever you do, blame and guilt will only make the situation worse. Even if it's very normal for your toddler to wake you up at 4 a.m. demanding blueberry pancakes, it's also not behavior that you want to reward or allow to continue.

Whatever concerning behaviors you're seeing in your child, the first step is to communicate with your co-parent and make a sincere effort to correct those behaviors in a healthy way. All of the advice given to you in this book is good, solid parenting advice that will help any kind of child to grow up happy and healthy. If your child's behaviors are truly cause for concern, you will see them start to ramp up when you start to change your responses. Even then, if you maintain consistency and commitment to your new parenting dynamic, you will most likely start to see those same behaviors taper off. Maintain contact with other important adults in your child's life, such as teachers and their pediatrician. Feel free to communicate with them which behaviors you're concerned about, and see what kind of feedback you get.

Perhaps the best way to tell if your child is truly a problem is how willing they are to hurt other people. Does your child's confidence or kindness come at the expense of others, and are their negative behaviors motivated by a need to punish or diminish those around them?

When It's Time to Get Professional Help

Personality disorders are all-pervasive. They affect cognitive, social, and even language skills. Therefore, if therapeutic intervention is necessary, it's most effective when implemented both early and consistently. The goal of professional intervention is to ensure that your child grows up to live a happy and self-confident life, as free as they can be from the damaging effects of the disorder.

NPD is particularly important to catch early because it's in the nature of the disorder for people who have it to refuse treatment as they get older. Someone who pathologically views themselves as right and perfect will find it almost impossible to accept that they have a psychological disorder or that they need any kind of help, professional or otherwise. Narcissists are unable to see or care about other people's perspectives, and so the damage their behavior does to others won't motivate them to seek help, either.

However, simply learning the common causes of NPD doesn't always enable you to catch warning signs in your child's behavior. The unfortunate reality is that NPD doesn't emerge from problematic parenting alone—there are a number of possible genetic and environmental causes that have been linked with the disorder. There are narcissists whose parents overvalued them and narcissists whose parents abused them. You and your co-parent are trying every positive parenting technique you can get your hands on, without success. When is it time to bring in a professional?

The maddening (but truthful) answer is that you'll know when it's the right time. In broad psychological terms, narcissism is actually a sub-form of sociopathy. This means that a truly narcissistic child will have heightened emotions, depression, and even criminal tendencies, especially when compared with the child's peers. No parent wants to see disorder and disturbance in their child, especially a child they love very much. So the fact that you picked up this book at all means that you at least suspect something may be wrong. And if you've made it this far into the book without feeling convinced that your child's behavior is just normal childhood narcissism, then there's no reason for you *not* to seek out professional help.

When evaluating for NPD, your therapist won't just be evaluating your child—they will be evaluating you and your co-parent, too. This can sound intimidating, but it will actually result in valuable feedback that you can use to improve your parenting style. This can only help your child, no matter their ultimate diagnosis. Even if your child doesn't have NPD, your therapist may discover that the behaviors you found so concerning are indicators of another problem.

If your child has started to actively bully or harm other children, including their siblings, that's a clear sign that it's time for an intervention. Antagonistic or abnormally aggressive behaviors indicate that your child has a problem with emotional intimacy. Their lack of empathy and need to be the center of attention is starting to impair their ability to relate to others. A chronic inability to maintain healthy social relationships is definitely a red flag and indicates that there is something (narcissism or otherwise) preventing your child from developing normal interpersonal skills.

These are the skills that they can learn from a therapist. Bringing your child to therapy, whether it's one-on-one or group, intentionally puts them in a safe environment where they can learn to manage their negative behaviors and resolve the underlying feelings that are causing them (Gross, 2015b). Even if there's "nothing wrong" with your child, everyone can benefit from therapeutic attention. There's no way that taking your child to see a therapist can harm or distort their development. Waiting to reach out when you suspect your child might be struggling, however, can have serious consequences in the future. Concerning behavior in children always has some underlying cause. A therapist can help you and your child get to the emotional root of their destructive behaviors and resolve those emotions so that they can move forward with their lives in a positive and healthy direction.

There is no cure for NPD. However, therapy can teach both you and your child healthy ways to manage the disorder. The actual diagnosis of NPD will take a long time to get and involve a lengthy evaluation that includes questionnaires, physical tests, and conversations with the therapist. Once the evaluation is complete, the therapist will come up with a mental health care plan that's specifically tailored to your child's needs and symptoms. The plan will likely include some form of therapy, a series of behaviors to practice at home or school and a targeted list of symptoms that the therapist feels need to be managed.

In therapy, your child will learn cognitive, communicative, and other skills that will enable them to recognize and resolve their destructive behaviors. Typically, the goal of therapy for people with narcissistic traits is to improve their self-esteem and teach them how to have more realistic expectations of other people. Narcissists at any stage of life can (and have) learned to relate to others in positive ways, but this largely depends on how open they are to feedback and how willing they are to act on that feedback (Nazario, 2020).

There are a few things that your therapist will look for in their initial evaluation. For starters, many symptoms of NPD overlap with other personality disorders. It's also possible to have more than one personality disorder, though this kind of determination is unlikely to be made for someone under the age of 18. When making an evaluation for NPD, your therapist will look for the general signs and symptoms of NPD as outlined in the DSM-5. They will also look for any physical or neurological conditions that may also explain your child's behavior. If necessary, the therapist may do an in-depth psychological evaluation using questionnaires and formal diagnostic tools like the NPI (*Narcissistic personality disorder - Diagnosis and treatment - Mayo Clinic*, 2017).

The only treatment available for NPD is psychotherapy. There are no medications that can treat the symptoms of narcissistic personality disorder. Medications will only be included in your child's treatment if the therapist suspects there may be another condition behind their behavior. They may also prescribe an antidepressant if your child shows signs of depression or anxiety.

In psychotherapy (otherwise known as talk therapy), your child will work one-on-one with a professional to learn why their behavior is destructive and learn better ways to cope with the emotions behind those behaviors. Psychotherapy will help your child better relate with other people, and therefore build relationships that are more intimate and enjoyable. It will also help them to understand what triggers their negative emotions and how to express those emotions without becoming competitive or distrusting of others.

The therapist will most likely devise a list of goals for your child to work toward, including the ability to accept and maintain intimate personal relationships, have a healthy and realistic idea of their competence, an increased ability to understand and recognize their feelings, recognize and better tolerate failure, and release their desire for unattainable goals.

The amount of time your child spends in therapy will depend on the severity of their initial symptoms, and how responsive they are to treatment and the ultimate goals outlined in their mental health care plan. Often, the therapist will recommend that you and your co-parent also participate in therapy of your own, either together with your child or independently with a parenting specialist.

Especially in the beginning, your child may feel defensive about going to therapy or insist that it's not necessary. It's in the nature of NPD to dislike self-reflection, and so the more pronounced your child's narcissistic traits, the more resistant they will be to professional intervention. Try to remain patient and supportive. Remind them to keep an open mind and focus on the rewards of going to therapy.

It's very important to make sure that your child does not miss any sessions. Remember, narcissists are incredibly manipulative. If you allow them to skip even one therapy visit, you're giving them the information they need to get out of therapy more often in the future.

If your child is struggling with drug or alcohol abuse, treatment for this should always take precedence over treatment for narcissism. Addictions and depression tend to feed off of one another, which is a dangerous combination for anyone. For narcissists, this can cause a serious amplification of narcissistic traits, which will make it almost impossible for them to face the reality of their addiction.

Preparing Yourself and Your Child for Your First Appointment

You've gone through the evaluation process, and you've been referred to a psychologist who will help your child. Before your first appointment, there are a few things you can do to help things move forward as smoothly as possible (*Narcissistic personality disorder - Diagnosis and treatment - Mayo Clinic,* 2017):

- Make a list of the symptoms you've seen in your child and how long they've been going on.
- Determine, as best you can, any possible causes or triggers for these behaviors, including traumatic past events or exposure to a narcissistic family member.
- Have your child's medical records handy, including information about any preexisting physical or psychological condition.
- Make a list of any medications your child may be taking, including the dosages.
- If possible, go with your co-parent or another trusted family member. This person can help take some of the pressure off of you, and if they know your child, they can potentially offer additional insight to the therapist.

Most importantly, make a list of any and all questions you wish to ask the psychologist. There is no question that's silly or stupid, so don't be afraid to ask anything that will help clarify things for you. To get you started, some questions you may wish to ask are:

- What type of disorder do you think my child may have?

- Could they have any other mental health conditions?
- What are the goals of this kind of therapy?
- Which kinds of therapy are most likely to be effective for my child?
- How much do you believe my child's quality of life can improve with therapy?
- How often will my child need to come to therapy, and how long do you expect treatment to last?
- Would family or group therapy be helpful for my child?
- Are there medications that can help my child manage their symptoms?
- My child has [other physical or mental health condition]. How will that impact my child's treatment?
- Are there any resources for parents that you can recommend for me? Is there any additional counseling or learning that you would suggest?

Your child's mental health provider may also ask you some questions to better understand your child's behavior, including:

- What are your child's symptoms?
- How long have these symptoms been going on, and what triggers them?

- How do these symptoms affect your child's life, including school or personal relationships?
- How does your child respond to criticism or rejection?
- Does your child have any close personal relationships? If not, what do you think is preventing them from making these kinds of connections?
- What are your child's major achievements or successes?
- Does your child have any goals or dreams for the future?
- Is your child able to recognize when someone else needs their help?
- How does your child respond when someone expresses difficult feelings?
- How would you describe the quality of your relationship with your child?
- Have any other family members been diagnosed with a mental health condition?
- Has your child been treated for any other mental health problems? Were any of these treatments effective?
- Does your child use alcohol or drugs?
- Is your child currently being treated for any physical or neurological conditions?

What Kinds of Treatments Are Available?

Not all therapy is the same. There are a few different therapeutic techniques that have been proven to have good results with narcissistic children and adults. In a general evaluation, the mental health provider will typically recommend a specific course of treatment that they believe will be effective for your child. However, you can also choose to research these different therapeutic styles on your own and reach out to therapists individually.

To give you a place to start, this is a simple guide to the different kinds of therapy typically recommended to people with narcissistic traits (Nair, 2018):

Cognitive Behavior Therapy

This is a one-on-one style of therapy. The therapist will work with your child to first help them recognize the problem. This will involve a variety of strategies that help your child identify their own negative behavior patterns. Over time, your child will begin to develop cognitive skills like emotional resilience, self-awareness, and the ability to label their feelings. These skills will help your child to better manage feelings of shame and anger and subsequently eliminate many of the triggers for their narcissism.

Psychoanalytic Psychotherapy

This kind of therapy will focus more on your child's grandiose self-image. The therapist will work with your child to help them see their defense mechanisms for what they are. Once your child is able to recognize their problematic behaviors as defensive strategies, they can then work with the therapist to improve their self-esteem and gain the interpersonal skills they need to improve the quality of their relationships. In this kind of therapy, counseling for the parents and family of the narcissistic child are often recommended as well.

Dialectical Behavior Therapy

This kind of therapy is most often recommended for covert and malignant narcissists. The therapist will work with your child to help them manage feelings of resentment and antagonism. More resilience against these feelings will then help your child to develop the interpersonal skills that their aggression had prevented them from learning in the past.

Group Therapy

In group therapy, your child will attend group sessions with other narcissists. This method has been found to be particularly effective with children, as it gives them valuable insight into what it's like to be on the receiving end of their destructive behaviors. This gives them a radical but valuable lesson in empathy and gives them the opportunity to practice healthy interpersonal skills with children who have similar social struggles.

Family Therapy

In family therapy, the entire family unit attends therapy sessions together. This helps the psychologist guide the family out of problematic dynamics that may be contributing to a child's narcissism. Since parenting has been found to have such a strong impact on the development of NPD, therapists will often recommend family therapy in addition to the child's individual treatment plan.

Chapter 6:

Relationships with Adult

Narcissistic Children

Parenting is a lifelong job. Whether your child is three or 30, you will still be concerned for their health and well-being and doing your best to guide them through the world. In the case of narcissistic "children," many parents don't realize that their child's narcissism is a problem until that child has reached young adulthood. Children's psychologists generally don't look for NPD, and so it's not typically something that's caught or addressed until the child reaches the minimum diagnostic age.

Adult children with narcissism can wreak a great deal of havoc on you and the rest of the family if their behavior remains unaddressed. Unlike with small children, adult narcissists rarely agree to get professional help or even admit that they have a problem, and so it often falls to the narcissist's loved ones to adopt strategies for self-protection. It can be very difficult to admit or accept that your child is a narcissist, but if you recognize any of the symptoms outlined in this book as applying to your adult child, then accepting the reality of your child's condition is the best thing you can do for yourself and for them.

That being said, adult narcissists rarely respond well to adjustments in your behavior, especially ones that benefit you and preserve your boundaries. You may find yourself faced with more unfair accusations and manipulations than ever before. If your child lives with you, setting healthy boundaries with them can feel like an impossible task. At the heart of it, you still love your child. How can you support them without sacrificing your own health to their needs?

The first step toward recovery is admitting that you need to recover. Your child may not be willing or able to hear that they have a problem and can be very skilled at convincing you that the things you do to heal yourself are harmful to them. And their threats aren't always empty—narcissists have the highest suicide rate of any personality disorder (Hammond, 2018b).

But once you have recognized your child's condition, however, you can take appropriate steps to minimize the damage caused by their behavior and try to build a relationship with them that is healthy for both of you. The same behaviors can manifest very differently in both adults and children, and so the strategies you need to protect yourself will be similar to the strategies for handling narcissistic children, but with some key adaptations for managing your adult child.

Give Affirmations

This is a proactive technique, something you can make a regular part of your interactions with your adult child, rather than something you do after an incident as damage control. Narcissists need a daily dose of attention and affection. Giving your child positive affirmations boosts their ego, which, in turn, gives them the attention that they crave. Affirmations make the narcissist feel noticed and secure, soothing their need to act out in destructive or manipulative ways. These affirmations don't have to be false or overdone. Think of the narcissist as an extra-sensitive child, one that needs to be recognized whenever they've done something well (which, in a way, is the truth).

Give Yourself a Break

Whenever you interact with the narcissist, make sure you have a private place that you can retreat to whenever the narcissist becomes too difficult or hurtful. Spending time with a narcissist can be incredibly emotionally draining. As with any job, spending long blocks of time with the narcissist will require regular breaks for you to rest and care for yourself. This strategy is especially important if the narcissist lives with you.

Start by giving yourself 15-minutes of private time in the morning and in the evening. This will give you a few moments alone to recover from their nasty words and allow you to think clearly about the right way to respond. Have several places available where you can be alone without fear of discovery or interruption. A common narcissistic abuse tactic is to create confusion. They challenge things that you know to be true or deny things that you witnessed happening. This makes you start to question yourself and your own inner voice, making the narcissist's voice the only one that you can hear. Giving yourself a break gives you the space you need to get the narcissist's influence out of your head and return to what you know to be true.

Allow Yourself to Recover

Coming to terms with your adult child's narcissism and the damage it may have caused throughout your life is not an easy process. It's important to give yourself the time and energy you need to recover from a lifetime of narcissistic manipulations. Sorting through years of the narcissist's abuses and the resulting trauma and releasing pent-up emotions or thoughts that you've never been able to express can be a long and painful process. As such, remember to be patient with yourself. Allow yourself to recover at a pace that is right for you. Seek out therapeutic assistance for yourself. Give yourself the space and time to heal so that you don't end up re-traumatizing yourself the next time you interact with the narcissist. All of this will ensure that the healing you do will be complete and have long-lasting effects.

Use Examples

Narcissists don't like to hear that their behavior is less than perfect. Rather than criticizing the narcissist directly, try referencing popular figures such as politicians or athletes who display the same narcissistic tendencies you see in your adult child. Express your dislike for those behaviors and even talk about how you would feel if your child behaved in that way. This can start to indirectly wake your adult child up to the realities of narcissistic dysfunction and even prompt them to discover narcissism as a condition on their own. This method is especially effective if you use someone that you know your child dislikes. If your child catches themselves behaving like an actor or politician that they hate, they'll quickly change their behavior to avoid being compared to someone they consider inferior.

Don't Respond to Threats

Threatening suicide is a very powerful manipulation tactic, one that narcissists use often. In the face of repeated suicidal threats, it's important to reach out for professional help. One of the ways a professional can help you is to create a contractual agreement between you, the narcissist, and the healthcare provider—one that allows for immediate, legal hospitalization the next time the narcissist threatens to kill themselves. If these threats are a manipulation strategy, the narcissist will likely stop in order to avoid the embarrassment of hospitalization. If you go this route, however, it's important to enforce the terms of the contract and call for hospitalization the next time your adult child threatens suicide.

Go to Family Therapy

Family therapy is an option for children and parents of all ages. If your adult child agrees to go to family therapy with you, invite your co-parent and/or other children to attend as well. The more people are in therapy with the narcissist, the easier it will be to keep everyone accountable for their own behavior.

Soften the Blow

Confronting narcissists outright is rarely effective. No matter how reasonably you approach them, they will likely feel attacked and therefore become too defensive to listen. Instead, try the "hamburger" method. This is a way to gently confront someone who is extremely sensitive to criticism or disagreements. The method is simple—give the other person a compliment, then offer a criticism, and then follow-up with a final compliment. Couching the criticism between two compliments will soften the criticism's impact and therefore increase the narcissist's ability to hear what you're saying.

Never Tolerate Abuse

Abuse is the number one reason that spouses divorce their narcissistic partners. If your narcissist starts to engage in behaviors that are outright abusive, you are never obligated to let them. Walk away, hang up the phone, or otherwise remove yourself from the situation the moment any abusive behaviors start to happen. If necessary, don't hesitate to block their calls or call the police. This sends the message to the narcissist that their old tactics will no longer be effective (Hammond, 2018b).

Protect against Gaslighting

The more abusive a narcissist is, the more likely they are to gaslight. Their denial of reality can both make you feel crazy and make it very difficult to reach out for help from other people. Record as many interactions with the narcissist as you possibly can. If you send them money, save the bank record. If you have an important conversation with them, take notes immediately afterwards or even record it if you can. Get them to say and do as many things on camera as you possibly can. Take screenshots of text messages or social media posts. All of this will give you something to reference if the narcissist starts to gaslight or deny reality.

Don't Lose Yourself

Narcissists view everyone around them as an inferior extension of themselves. When constantly interacting with someone who treats you this way, it's very easy to believe them. Don't allow the narcissist to convince you that your own, unique identity is not valid, or that your needs, life, and emotions are not as valuable as theirs. Don't allow them to tell you who you are or convince you that they know you better than you know yourself. They don't.

Beware of Crumbs

Remember, crumbs are brief moments when the child appears to be complying with your wishes for their behavior. These moments are very common in adult narcissistic children, and when they happen, it's tempting to see them as a glimpse of their old self coming up through the narcissistic persona. But don't allow yourself to be fooled. Your adult child's narcissistic behavior, for better or for worse, has become part of who they are. If your adult child is briefly behaving the way you wish they would, it's most likely a manipulative tactic. Once they get what they want from you, they'll revert back to their narcissistic ways.

The chances of an adult narcissist permanently changing their behavior is very slim, for the simple reason that they would have to recognize that they have a problem in order to seek professional help. When interacting with an adult narcissist, it's best to accept them for who they are, and avoid the temptation to long for the person they were before their narcissistic tendencies emerged. Instead, if you wish to maintain your relationship with the narcissist, you'll need to engage in strategies that protect you from their abusive behavior.

Establish a Connection with their Spouse

If your child gets married, warning their spouse about your child's narcissism may seem like the responsible thing to do. Unfortunately, this will only serve to make you seem like *you're* the one who's manipulative or interfering and give the narcissist the evidence they need to smear your name or alienate you from the rest of the family. Instead, make yourself available to your child's spouse. Be there for them if they have any questions. Try to establish a healthy relationship with them, just as you would if your child wasn't a narcissist. Above all, believe them if they start to tell you stories about your child's behavior at home.

Do What You Can For Their Children

All too often, grandchildren become just another weapon that the narcissist can use to manipulate, punish, and otherwise control your behavior. Your narcissistic adult child may prevent you from seeing your grandchildren. They may also insist that you are hurting your grandchildren by not doing what the narcissist wants. As confusing and hurtful as this can be, don't allow the narcissist to use their children in this way. Instead, maintain the boundaries that you have with them. When you do see your grandchildren, build a healthy relationship with them so that you can become a grounding and positive force in their lives.

Go to Therapy

Getting therapy yourself can be a critical part of both recovery and management of your relationship with your narcissistic child. A therapist can help you to heal from past or present wounds, let go of destructive feelings, and give strategies for resolving stressful dynamics with the narcissist. If the narcissist's behaviors become extremely toxic, the therapist can also support you through the decision to distance yourself from your adult child and the subsequent grief you feel afterward.

All of these strategies are effective with adult narcissists, and they can be critically important for you if you are living with one. Employing these in your daily interactions will help you to establish healthy boundaries and therefore lessen the control the narcissist has over your life. If you ever feel unsafe or overwhelmed, don't hesitate to reach out to professional sources for help. If you cannot seem to manage your relationship with your child in a healthy way, there is one last option available to you.

Going No-Contact

If things become truly dangerous for you and/or other members of the family, you may have no choice but to cease all contact with the narcissist. It can be deeply painful for a parent to tell their child that they no longer wish to see them anymore, but the alternative is to spend a lifetime suffering their abuses and never building a loving relationship with them. Worse, your inability to cut the narcissist out of your life could harm other members of the family, including your co-parent and the narcissist's siblings.

If you go this route, commit to it completely. You may have to remove pictures or objects that bring up painful memories or feelings, at least until you have had a chance to grieve and recover from your loss. If other people in the family remain in contact with the narcissist, resist the urge to talk about them or get updates about their lives. You will not be able to recover fully from the damaging effects of the narcissist's influence if you are longing for better times in the past or hanging on to the hope that the narcissist will somehow learn from their mistakes. There's always the possibility to reestablish contact in the future, but you cannot make a clean, healthy break from the narcissist's toxic influence if you are dependent on this possibility to get you through the grieving process.

A less intense version of going no-contact is to severely distance yourself from the narcissist. Do not allow them to live with you. Limit the time you spend talking on the phone, and ignore any phone calls or text messages that violate your boundaries. Do not follow them on social media, and if they use this as a way to manipulate or abuse you, block them on those platforms. Limit visits to holidays or other key events where there will be lots of other family members around, and avoid spending one-on-one time with them as much as you can.

Going No-Contact

Ending your relationship with your child is obviously a last resort and an option that parents take when they have no other choice. No matter how bad things have gotten with your child, this decision can still be an incredibly difficult and painful one to make. To cope, many parents report thinking of their children as dead (Narcissist Abuse Support, 2019b).

The grief that parents experience after going no-contact with their children is very real. This is a termination of the relationship, and the choice is made with the understanding that you might never see your child again. Narcissists take up so much of your time and energy that it can be extremely disorienting to suddenly experience life without them. Their tendency to damage your sense of identity can leave you feeling like you don't know who you are without them.

As such, it's very important to get therapy for yourself after ceasing contact with your child. A therapist can help you through the grieving process, as well as help you to rediscover yourself without the narcissist's destructive influence. After so many years of abuse, some parents report feelings of numbness toward their child, and so a therapist can help you to re-access your feelings of love for your child in a safe and supportive environment.

A therapist can also give you the support you need when confronted with triggers or painful memories during the grieving process. They can help you to live in a house that you may have shared with your child, get through holidays or other significant events, and eliminate triggering pictures or objects from your home. If other people in the family are still in contact with the narcissist, a therapist can help you to navigate conversations with those family members and set boundaries with them that protect your decision not to see them anymore.

The painful truth is that the future of a narcissistic child is not a hopeful one. Their destructive behavior will make it difficult to keep anyone in their lives for very long. You may be the first in the family to distance yourself, but it will only be a matter of time before other members of the family do the same. No matter how many people choose to leave them, many narcissists are never able to face the reality that their own behavior is what's damaging their relationships. Over and over again, it will be the fault of the person who leaves them. Sometimes, the fact that others have gone no-contact becomes a manipulative tool that they use in the future, regaling others with stories of how their family "abandoned" them.

If you choose to go no-contact, don't allow yourself to believe that you have abandoned your child. No matter the severity of their disorder, every adult is responsible for their own actions. If your child is causing harm to you or anyone else, then you are absolutely within your rights to do what you need to do to protect yourself and other members of the family.

You may have heard the advice that in order to love others, you must first learn to love yourself. This advice certainly rings true for narcissists. It applies to the people who are close to them as well. Instead of viewing your choice to go no-contact as an act of aggression towards your child, try to see it as an act of love for yourself. Freeing yourself from the narcissist's toxic influence may be the only thing you can do to recover and start to develop new, healthy relationships. Part of the recovery process will be learning how to prevent yourself from getting into relationships with narcissists in the future, as well as learning how to manage triggers that remind you of your child's past abuses.

Without the narcissist's veil of lies and control, you'll start to realize that the world is a much more fun and interesting place when you are allowed to be yourself and make your own decisions. You will need to find new activities that help you to rediscover both the world and your unique place in it. Your past relationship with your child almost certainly damaged your sense of identity and personal boundaries. A major part of narcissistic abuse recovery is actively participating in activities that help you to restore your sense of control and your trust in yourself.

The ultimate goal of recovery is for you to reclaim what the narcissist in your life took from you. You will need to learn how to build relationships in which reciprocation is not only available, but valued. You may also have to repair damaged relationships with other people in your home or neighborhood as you take steps to slowly rebuild your boundaries.

Relationships with narcissists destroy your sense of self, and so, in the time after you've ceased contact, you'll need to actively reconstruct your lost identity. This involves both recognizing the ways in which your identity was stifled and then taking active steps to reconstruct it. With a narcissist in your life, your world begins to revolve around the narcissist. Without them, you will have to reenter the world and learn how to reorder your life with yourself at the center.

Narcissistic loved ones slowly but surely chip away at the lines between your needs and theirs. Their inability to self-reflect sabotages your ability to do the same. Your ability to turn inward or have any sense of independent self-hood is systematically destroyed, as the narcissist cannot tolerate moments when your full attention isn't focused on them. Once you've distanced yourself from this toxic influence, you will be free to once again honor your own self-awareness. By the time you are driven to cease contact with someone, your life has been consumed with them and their needs for a damagingly long time. Many parents have to relearn how to self-reflect and think about themselves as having an independent identity.

On this journey of self-rediscovery, it's important that you neither get lost in introspection or start looking desperately for new relationships to fill the void left by the narcissist. It's very common for parents to feel empty and lost after distancing themselves from a narcissistic child. The guidance of a therapist can help you to see that this feeling of emptiness was exactly what your child wanted. They systematically emptied you so that you would pour all of your time, energy, and resources into them and their needs. Without them, you are tasked with once again finding meaning and substance in your life without becoming narcissistic yourself. In recovery, you'll learn how to balance taking care of yourself and taking care of others. You'll learn how to put yourself first without harming others. The only way to do this is to fully accept that your relationship with your child was indeed abusive. Accepting this truth will give you the ability to finally face reality, something that your narcissistic child may never be able to do.

Even choosing to distance yourself without cutting off contact entirely gives you the valuable space you need to realize who you are and what role you play in your child's life. Do you act like your true self around your child? Do you even understand how you act, or how your relationship with the narcissist has impacted other members of the family?

Narcissistic abuse leaves a specific kind of trauma, one that manifests in a few specific ways (Covert, 2020):

Low Self-Esteem

By the time you establish no-contact with your child, your sense of self will have been severely damaged. Much of the critical work done in therapy is centered around recovering your sense of self, as this is the most difficult aspect of narcissistic abuse to overcome. Years and years living with unreasonable demands and verbal abuses will inevitably take their toll on a person. You may begin to feel that you are somehow not worthy of being loved or cared for. Recovering your self-esteem often involves therapeutic strategies that rekindle your lost belief in your own talents and abilities.

Anxiety

People in close relationships with narcissists live in a constant state of fear. You may go to great lengths to avoid upsetting your child. You fear the inevitable consequences of their anger and displeasure. This makes the child an omnipresent figure in the parent's life. Everything they do is done in hopes that it won't offend or upset the narcissistic child. They lack any kind of privacy or boundaries and if their child lives at home, find themselves without any ability to live a private life. Even after you've gone no-contact with your child and freed yourself from this dynamic, the fear will still remain with you as chronic anxiety and even post-traumatic stress disorder.

Self-Blame

Parents of narcissistic children tend to blame themselves for the person their child grew to become. Even after going no-contact, many parents live with deep feelings of shame, viewing their need to cut off contact with their own child as a reflection on their poor parenting skills. In recovery, you will slowly begin to accept that your child's abuse was not your fault and that their personality disorder was something that developed without your knowledge or control.

Relationships of all kinds are an important vehicle for personal growth. Healthy relationships teach us valuable lessons about who we are, who we want to be, and what kind of influence we have on the world. In narcissistic relationships, however, these lessons are distorted. The parents of narcissistic children often become codependent, as this is typically the only way to sustain the relationship. The more codependent you are, the more toxic your relationship with your child becomes.

Empathic people are particularly vulnerable to narcissistic manipulations. In many ways, empaths are the opposite of narcissists, developing empathetic skills early in life that are advanced for their age-level. Unlike narcissists, empaths are highly sensitive to the needs and energies of the people around them. However, empaths can easily slip into codependency because they are so attuned to other people's problems that they start to absorb them as their own.

If you have a natural tendency to absorb or take on other people's emotions, you may be an empath yourself. Empaths are highly sensitive and intuitive, qualities that normally enhance the quality of their relationships. However, because they are so sensitive, empaths can sometimes struggle to verbally express or articulate their feelings. Ironically, they have the same trouble with boundaries that narcissists have, but inverted—they have trouble laying boundaries because they are *so* sensitive to other people's feelings. For example, if someone around them is feeling depressed or anxious, they start to feel depressed and anxious, too. This creates the perfect situation for a narcissist. The empath gives the narcissist all the attention and sympathy that the narcissist craves and is so attuned to the narcissist's emotions that they mirror the narcissist's own feelings back to them, which only encourages their narcissism. When this kind of dynamic reaches pathological levels, the empath graduates from a healthy level of empathy to codependency.

If you took the NPI after reading about it in Chapter 1 and got a score of 10 or below, you are most likely codependent. Codependency is not a personality disorder, but it is a very real pattern of behavior that causes the codependent to care for the needs and feelings of their loved ones with toxically low regard for their own feelings. Codependency is complex enough to merit its own book, but it's worth mentioning here because it's very common for people in close relationships with narcissists to become codependent. Codependents feel incapable and unworthy unless they are actively helping other people. Narcissists prey on these feelings, weaponizing the codependent's lack of self-esteem in order to feed their own ego.

Whether you've developed codependent behaviors or not, narcissistic relationships can be extremely toxic. Narcissistic relationships with children can be extremely difficult because their destructive behaviors typically arise out of normal childhood narcissism or a problematic childhood (which may not have been within your control to prevent). No matter how it begins, the narcissistic child learns that they can manipulate their parents and other family members to satisfy their own need for personal glorification. In order to keep the peace, family members either develop strained and distant relationships with the narcissist or develop codependent tendencies in order to survive the narcissist's abuse. Narcissists use the same tactics in all of their relationships, which makes them more volatile than other kinds of abusers who are able to contain or target their abusive behavior.

Narcissistic children begin life the way all children do—by idolizing their parents. Narcissistic adults are people who never grew out of this idolization. Though it certainly may not feel like it, narcissistic children can behave as savagely as they do because they put their parents on a pedestal. In a way, controlling you is the ultimate victory for them because you are such a powerful figure in their subconscious.

The relationship between parent and narcissistic child is unique because your child doesn't have to do any work to charm you or win your affections. The more pronounced their narcissism becomes, the more they start to realize how difficult it is for you to judge their behavior objectively. They prey on your natural parental instincts to forgive and protect them, warping the unconditional love of a parent into a toxic and abusive dynamic. It's difficult for parents to discern the difference between normal childhood behavior and toxic narcissistic displays. The more codependent you become with the narcissist, the less able you are to hear any negative criticism of your child's behaviors, even if they deeply hurt you. You may even start to defend or deny their behaviors to others, further justifying and protecting them from negative consequences. This forges a special bond between the narcissist and their parents because parents are often the very last relationships they have left after everyone else in their life has distanced themselves.

Adult narcissistic children can be extremely obsessive and emotionally needy. They will go to great lengths to keep you focused on them at all times, including bursting into tears or even threatening suicide. These tactics can be incredibly difficult to see through and are often successful in preventing you from having any kind of healthy life. If they aren't married, narcissists are very likely to live with their parents, as this further erodes the boundaries between them. The tantrums, rages, and verbal attacks that you became used to in childhood never go away but continue long into their adult life. In adults, these rages can quickly become abusive, either verbally or even physically. Often, the child will then make a great show of guilt and remorse after these explosive episodes. These dramatic displays convince you to forgive their behavior or even start to believe that it was somehow your fault. And before you know it, the behavior has repeated itself all over again.

If and when you start to lay boundaries or see their behavior for the abuse that it is, the narcissist will quickly change their tactics. They may become more manipulative or start gaslighting you into believing that their abusive behavior isn't that bad. Adult narcissists are much more skilled at deceptive tactics than narcissistic children, a feature of NPD that makes it particularly difficult to handle in adults. Your child may change their behavior so fluidly that it can be difficult to identify their true feelings or personality. This confusion is intentional and meant to keep your attention focused solely on them. When their lies and deceptions collapse, they lash out in anger, engage in pathological denial, or gaslight you into questioning your reality.

The Cycle of Narcissistic Abuse

When your relationship reaches an abusive level, going no-contact may be the only choice you have to live a happy and healthy life.

Abusive relationships with narcissists typically cycle back and forth between two distinct stages (Covert, 2020):

   1.   *Love-Bombing*

In romantic relationships, this is sometimes called the "honeymoon" stage. This is the narcissist at their most charming. They may get you (the parent) an extravagant gift for Christmas or write you a deeply moving card for your birthday. They will do whatever you want or need, going to levels that your co-parent or other children won't even go to in order to help you or make you comfortable. They may tell you frequently that they love you or wish you could be more actively involved in their life somehow. If they don't live with you, they may tell you that they miss you or start texting you all the time. Perhaps they invite you out to eat or start making grand plans about a vacation they'd like to take with you in the future. Maybe they offer to paint your bedroom walls or encourage you to try something new. They may start openly inviting you to participate in your life in ways that they didn't before, such as zooming with the grandchildren or inviting you to their church.

In this stage, the narcissist is extremely fun, warm, and enjoyable to be around. They will share all their hopes and dreams with you. They may even seem to take an interest in yours. Even if their attention feels overwhelming or over-the-top, you can't help but appreciate the apparent effort that they're making to connect with you. Favors that seem like "too much" might be a bit stressful, but appreciated. After all, how can you be unhappy that your child wants to spend time with you?

It's the return to this stage that often convinces parents to stay trapped in abusive relationships, as they become convinced that this is the "true" child, and their destructive behavior is just some kind of darkness they have to overcome.

2. *Devaluation*

The charming, loving stage can last a few weeks or even a few months at a time. It lasts just long enough to convince you that your child is inherently loving and that if you can just show them how much you love them back, all of their narcissistic behaviors will simply go away. Sadly, this is not the reality of the situation. Once you become comfortable enough to start relaxing and turning your attention back to your own life, the narcissist suddenly changes from over-attentive golden child to enraged abuser.

This stage can begin gradually or happen suddenly. Some narcissists start to slowly withdraw their kindnesses or displays of affection. They may become moody or stop returning your calls. Over time, this will start to confuse you and ultimately lead you to believe that this change was triggered by something you did or said. Everything was going so well before. What changed?

Sometimes, the devaluation stage will begin suddenly and without warning. A perceived slight or the laying of a boundary can cause the narcissist to fly into a rage. It can often feel like a switch was flipped, and the child you know and love was suddenly replaced with a destructive monster. All of a sudden, nothing you do is appreciated and everything you do is wrong. They start to criticize everything about you. They may make snide comments about your friends or other members of the family. They may actively seek to humiliate you in front of other members of the family in an attempt to alienate you from them. They may find fault in your appearance or lifestyle. Anything that may make you outshine them or that they didn't personally approve of will be attacked and condemned.

Typically, your response to this stage will be to do whatever you can to appease the narcissist's wrath. When they revert back to the love-bombing stage, you'll feel as though you and your child have somehow made progress, and the cycle begins all over again.

Conclusion

Narcissism is not a diagnosis that many parents want to hear for their child. After reading through the more severe descriptions of NPD and its symptoms in this book, you may be feeling a bit apprehensive about getting help for your own child.

But don't let the popular connotations around this word scare you. Moving forward, there are a few key things to remember that will keep you focused on recovery and a positive journey forward for yourself and your child.

First, you now know that all children under the age of 18 display narcissistic characteristics. Not only is this no cause for alarm, it's actually a sign that your child is developing in a healthy way. It's for this reason that most psychologists are very hesitant to diagnose children with narcissism, as it can create a false sense of concern around what are relatively normal and age-appropriate behaviors. If none of the more severe symptoms of narcissism ring true for your child, then you can rest assured that all your child needs is some love and guidance from you to grow into a happy and healthy adult. The parenting techniques you learned in this book will benefit children of all kinds, not just narcissistic ones.

Second, there's a big difference between being narcissistic and having narcissistic personality disorder, or NPD. Throughout this book, I have sometimes used these terms interchangeably. However, it's diagnostically impossible for children to actually have NPD. So if your child *is* displaying some concerning symptoms, the good news is that you've caught those symptoms in time. The earlier you can recognize your child's problematic behaviors and learn how to correct them, the less likely your child will be to develop a personality disorder later in life. Narcissism is no better or worse a diagnosis than any other. As with any other mental health condition your child might have, as soon as you start to notice problematic symptoms, you do what you can to help your child learn to manage them.

Don't hesitate to reach out for professional help. Therapy can seem intimidating to some, especially for parents who did not go to therapy when they were children. You'll probably find that there's a big difference between therapy for adults and therapy for kids. Psychologists who work with children have spent years learning how to make their treatments fun and age-appropriate. Think of your child's psychologist the same way you think about their teachers at school or their pediatrician or their dentist. This is just another professional in your child's life that's going to help you give that child the best possible chance at a happy life.

Last, but certainly not least, do not give up hope if your child does develop NPD or if you are concerned for an adult child whose symptoms are quite severe. There are many people with NPD who learn how to live happy and fulfilling lives. There are people who have learned how to cope with the narcissist's more problematic behaviors in ways that are healthy and beneficial for everyone. Like any other disorder, learn how to modify your interactions with your child in order to best support both their health and yours. If you do have to resort to going no-contact, know that there are many resources out there for people who survived abusive relationships with narcissistic loved ones.

My sincere hope for this book is that it gives you the insight you need to recognize the narcissist in your life, whether it be your child, your co-parent, or even your own parents. Simply learning to see narcissism for what it is can go a long way toward empowering you to navigate those relationships in a safer and healthier way. My intention with this book is not to scare you but to make you feel more secure in your ability to manage your child's narcissism in an appropriate way. No matter how old your child is or what kinds of symptoms they display, it's never too late for them to get help. My hope is that this book sets you on a path toward positive outcomes, both for yourself and for your child. You now have all the resources you need to begin working towards recovery and healing, towards an improved family dynamic, and, above all, an improved relationship with the child you love so much.

If you enjoyed this book or gained any valuable insight from it, please leave a review on Amazon! Your feedback helps me to produce better content in the future and will help other concerned parents decide if this is the right book for them.

References

Arabi, S. (2020, July 12). *20 Diversion Tactics Highly Manipulative Narcissists, Sociopaths And Psychopaths Use To Silence You.* Thought Catalog. https://thoughtcatalog.com/shahida-arabi/2016/06/20-diversion-tactics-highly-manipulative-narcissists-sociopaths-and-psychopaths-use-to-silence-you/

Bash, A. (2017). *Narcissistic Siblings and the Pain You Feel from Them.* Families. https://vocal.media/families/narcissistic-siblings-and-the-pain-you-feel-from-them

Bergeron, N. C. (2019, November 7). *Inside The Narcissist's Mind, And How We Invite Them Into Our Lives.* C. Nathan Bergeron. https://cnathanbergeron.com/inside-narcissists-mind-invite-lives/

Bridges to Recovery. (2020, October 25). *A One-Sided Rivalry: The Traumatic Effects of Narcissistic Personality Disorder on Siblings.* https://www.bridgestorecovery.com/blog/a-one-sided-rivalry-the-traumatic-effects-of-narcissistic-personality-disorder-on-siblings/

Covert, J. D. (2019). *Divorcing and Healing from a Narcissist: Emotional and Narcissistic Abuse Recovery. Co-parenting after an Emotionally destructive Marriage*

and Splitting up with a toxic ex. Independently
published.

Cunha, J. (2020, August 10). *What Are the Signs of a*
Narcissistic Child? EMedicineHealth.
https://www.emedicinehealth.com/what_are_t
he_signs_of_a_narcissistic_child/article_em.ht
m

Dawson, M. (2015, March 25). *How not to raise a narcissist*
in 9 easy steps. New York Post.
https://nypost.com/2015/03/11/how-not-to-
raise-a-narcissist-in-9-easy-steps/

Firestone, L. (2019, January 17). *What Really Goes On in*
the Mind of a Narcissist? PsychAlive.

https://www.psychalive.org/what-really-goes-on-in-the-mind-of-a-narcissist/

Foster, J. D., Shiverdecker, L. K., & Turner, I. N. (2016, January 20). *What Does the Narcissistic Personality Inventory Measure Across the Total Score Continuum?* Current Psychology. https://link.springer.com/article/10.1007/s121 44-016-9407- 5?error=cookies_not_supported&code=a81d76 f9-3fc7-46a0-80f1-bd7cf45108d2

Frazier, B. (2015). *10 Strategies to Avoid Raising a Narcissist.* Thesuccessfulparent.Com. http://www.thesuccessfulparent.com/categorie s/moral-development/item/10-strategies-to-avoid-raising-a-narcissist#.X92MwdHYq3B

Gnaulati, E. (2013, September 17). *ADHD, or Childhood Narcissism?* The Atlantic. https://www.theatlantic.com/health/archive/2013/09/adhd-or-childhood-narcissism/279660/

Greenberg, E. (2017, October 26). *How children grow up to be narcissists.* Business Insider. https://www.businessinsider.com/how-children-grow-up-to-be-narcissists-2017-10?international=true&r=US&IR=T#scenario-2-the-devaluing-narcissistic-parent-2

Greenberg, E. (2020). *What Three Factors Predict if A Child Will Become a Narcissist?* Psychologytoday.Com. https://www.psychologytoday.com/intl/blog/

understanding-narcissism/202001/what-three-factors-predict-if-child-will-become-narcissist

Gross, G. (2015a, March 13). *Narcissism in children has many causes, but it can be addressed.* Washington Post.
https://www.washingtonpost.com/news/to-your-health/wp/2015/03/13/narcissism-in-children-has-many-causes-but-it-can-be-addressed/

Gross, G. (2015b, March 13). *Narcissism in children has many causes, but it can be addressed.* Washington Post.
https://www.washingtonpost.com/news/to-your-health/wp/2015/03/13/narcissism-in-

children-has-many-causes-but-it-can-be-
addressed/

Hamaker, S. (2015, March 11). *7 ways to nip narcissism in
the bud.* Washington Post.
https://www.washingtonpost.com/news/paren
ting/wp/2015/03/11/7-ways-to-nip-
narcissism-in-the-bud/

Hammond, M. C. S. (2016, December 10). *Is My Child
A Narcissist?* Psych Central.
https://www.psychcentral.com/pro/exhausted-
woman/2016/12/is-my-child-a-narcissist#1

Hammond, M. C. S. (2018a, March 23). *The Narcissistic
Cycle of Abuse Among Siblings.* Psych Central.
https://www.psychcentral.com/pro/exhausted-

woman/2018/03/the-narcissistic-cycle-of-
abuse-amoungst-siblings#1

Hammond, M. C. S. (2018b, August 31). *10 Strategies for
Coping with an Adult Narcissistic Child.* Psych
Central.
https://www.psychcentral.com/pro/exhausted-
woman/2018/08/10-strategies-for-coping-
with-an-adult-narcissistic-child#1

Hammond, M. C. S. (2019a, June 28). *Is My Child A
Narcissist?* The Exhausted Woman.
https://pro.psychcentral.com/exhausted-
woman/2016/12/is-my-child-a-narcissist/

Hammond, M. C. S. (2019b, June 29). *The Dysfunctional
Ways a Family Protects a Narcissist.* The Exhausted

Woman.

https://pro.psychcentral.com/exhausted-woman/2017/07/the-dysfunctional-ways-a-family-protects-a-narcissist/

How To Deal With A Child With Narcissistic Personality Disorder. (2019, December 3). [Video]. YouTube. https://www.youtube.com/watch?v=_Wed6u2RhVg

Jana, S. (2014, August 7). *https://search.google.com/structured-data/testing-tool/83780.* MomJunction. https://www.momjunction.com/articles/unexpected-treatments-for-narcissistic-personality-disorder-in-your-kid_0083780/

Johnson, B. (2017). *Childhood Roots of Narcissistic Personality Disorder.* Psychologytoday.Com. https://www.psychologytoday.com/us/blog/warning-signs-parents/201701/childhood-roots-narcissistic-personality-disorder

Just One Simple Question Can Identify Narcissistic People. (2014). News.Osu.Edu. https://news.osu.edu/just-one-simple-question-can-identify-narcissistic-people/

Krauss Whitbourne, S. (2020). *How Narcissists Protect Themselves from Feeling Like Losers.* Psychologytoday.Com. https://www.psychologytoday.com/us/blog/fulfillment-any-age/202011/how-narcissists-protect-themselves-feeling-losers

Lancer, D. (2019). *How to Think Like a Narcissist and Why They Hurt People*. Psychologytoday.Com. https://www.psychologytoday.com/us/blog/toxic-relationships/201906/how-think-narcissist-and-why-they-hurt-people

Lancer, J. D. D. (2020, June 5). *4 Types of Narcissism Share This Trait*. Psych Central. https://psychcentral.com/lib/4-types-of-narcissism-share-this-trait/

Morin, A. (2020). *15 Ways to Deal With a Narcissistic Teenage Daughter*. Verywell Family. https://www.verywellfamily.com/how-to-deal-with-a-narcissistic-teenage-daughter-4126480

Nair, A. (2018, October 26). *Narcissism in Children -*
Causes, Signs and Treatment. FirstCry Parenting.
https://parenting.firstcry.com/articles/narcissis
m-in-children-causes-signs-and-treatment/

Narcissism. (n.d.). Psychologytoday.Com.
https://www.psychologytoday.com/us/basics/
narcissism

Narcissist Abuse Support. (2019a, November 16).
Narcissistic Brother and Sister Sibling Traits - Start
Healing - Free eBook.
https://narcissistabusesupport.com/how-to-
identify-narcissistic-siblings-narcissistic-brother-
sister/

Narcissist Abuse Support. (2019b, December 11). *Do you think your child might be a narcissist? Young or old what to do?* https://narcissistabusesupport.com/i-think-my-child-is-a-narcissist-what-do-i-do/

Narcissistic personality disorder - Diagnosis and treatment - Mayo Clinic. (2017, November 18). Mayoclinic.Org. https://www.mayoclinic.org/diseases-conditions/narcissistic-personality-disorder/diagnosis-treatment/drc-20366690

Narcissistic personality disorder - Symptoms and causes. (2017, November 18). Mayo Clinic. https://www.mayoclinic.org/diseases-conditions/narcissistic-personality-

disorder/symptoms-causes/syc-20366662

Nazario, B. (2020). *What are treatments for narcissistic

personality disorder?* WebMD.

https://www.webmd.com/mental-

health/qa/what-are-treatments-for-narcissistic-

personality-disorder

Neuharth, D. (2019). *Seven Hidden Principles That Motivate

Narcissists.* Psychologytoday.Com.

https://www.psychologytoday.com/us/blog/n

arcissism-demystified/201905/7-hidden-

principles-motivate-narcissists

Ni, P. (2017). *Six Common Traits of Narcissists and

Gaslighters.* Psychologytoday.Com.

https://www.psychologytoday.com/intl/blog/communication-success/201707/6-common-traits-narcissists-and-gaslighters

Ni, P. (2019). *Seven Ways Narcissists Manipulate Relationships*. Psychologytoday.Com. https://www.psychologytoday.com/us/blog/communication-success/201903/7-ways-narcissists-manipulate-relationships

Psych Central Research Team. (2020, June 2). *Narcissistic Personality Quiz | Psych Central*. Psychology Tests & Quizzes. https://psychcentral.com/quizzes/narcissistic-personality-quiz/

Soeiro, L. (2019). *Four Types of Narcissist and How to Spot Each One*. Psychologytoday.Com. https://www.psychologytoday.com/us/blog/i-hear-you/201904/4-types-narcissist-and-how-spot-each-one

Specialist, T. T. (2020, April 20). *Parenting A Narcissistic Child or Teen*. The Treatment Specialist. https://thetreatmentspecialist.com/parenting-a-narcissistic-child/

Stines, S. (2019). *Common Traits of Narcissists*. Pro.Psychcentral.Com. https://pro.psychcentral.com/recovery-expert/2019/12/common-traits-of-narcissists/

van Schie, C. C., Jarman, H. L., Huxley, E., & Grenyer, B. F. S. (2020). Narcissistic traits in young people: understanding the role of parenting and maltreatment. *Borderline Personality Disorder and Emotion Dysregulation*, *7*(1), 7–10. https://doi.org/10.1186/s40479-020-00125-7

Walansky, A. (2020, November 25). *Narcissistic Children Have Parents Who Do These Things--How Not To Raise A Narcissist*. Goalcast. https://www.goalcast.com/2020/08/27/narcissistic-children-parenting-style-mistakes/

Webber, R. (2016). *Meet the Real Narcissists (They're Not What You Think*. Psychologytoday.Com. https://www.psychologytoday.com/us/articles

/201609/meet-the-real-narcissists-theyre-not-

what-you-think

Zeigler-Hill, V. (2019). *Inside the Mind of the Narcissist.*

Spsp.Org. https://www.spsp.org/news-

center/blog/zeigler-hill-narcissist

CPSIA information can be obtained
at www.ICGtesting.com
Printed in the USA
LVHW081930120822
725729LV00007BA/307

9 781087 943855